Practicing Hope

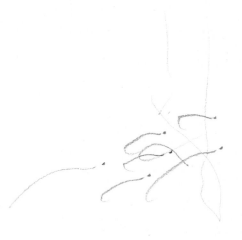

Select Titles in the EHAIA Series
Ecumenical HIV and AIDS Initiative in Africa
From the World Council of Churches

Compassionate Circles:
African Women Theologians
  Facing HIV
Edited by Ezra Chitando and
  Nontando Hadebe, 2009

Troubled but Not Destroyed:
African Theology in Dialogue with
  HIV and AIDS
Ezra Chitando, 2009

A Window into Hope:
An Invitation to Faith
  in the Context of HIV and AIDS
Robert Igo, o.s.b. 2009

Living with Hope:
African Churches and HIV/AIDS, 1
Ezra Chitando, 2007

Acting in Hope:
African Churches and HIV/AIDS, 2
Ezra Chitando, 2007

Beacons of Hope:
HIV Competent Churches—
  A Framework for Action
Sue Parry, 2008

Into the Sunshine:
Integrating HIV/AIDS in the Ethics
  Curriculum
Edited by Charles Kaagba and
  C. B. Peter, 2005

Africa Praying:
A Handbook on HIV/AIDS Sensitive
  Sermon Guidelines and Liturgy
Edited by Musa W. Dube, 2003

Listening with Love:
Pastoral Counselling—A Christian
  Response to People Living with
  HIV/AIDS
Robert Igo, o.s.b., 2005

HIV/AIDS and the Curriculum:
Methods of Integrating HIV/AIDS
  in Theological Programmes
Edited by Musa W. Dube, 2003

Practicing Hope
A Handbook for Building HIV and AIDS
Competence in the Churches

Sue Parry

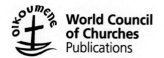

**World Council
of Churches**
Publications

Show me Your ways, O LORD
Teach me Your paths; guide me
In Your truth and teach me, for
You are my God, my Saviour, and my
Hope is in You all day long.
—Psalm 25:4-5

PRACTICING HOPE
A Handbook for Building HIV and AIDS Competence in the Churches
EHAIA series

WCC Publications is the book publishing programme of the World Council of Churches. Founded in 1948, the WCC promotes Christian unity in faith, witness and service for a just and peaceful world. A global fellowship, the WCC brings together more than 349 Protestant, Orthodox, Anglican and other churches representing more than 560 million Christians in 110 countries and works cooperatively with the Roman Catholic Church.

Opinions expressed in WCC Publications are those of the authors.

Scripture quotations, unless otherwise noted, are from the New Revised Standard Version Bible, © copyright 1989 by the Division of Christian Education of the National Council of the Churches of Christ in the USA. Used by permission.

Cover design: Adele Robey/Phoenix Graphics, Inc.

ISBN: 978-2-8254-1622-8

World Council of Churches
150 route de Ferney, P.O. Box 2100
1211 Geneva 2, Switzerland
http://publications.oikoumene.org

CONTENTS

INTRODUCTION

> HIV and AIDS constitute a global emergency, pose one of the
> most formidable challenges to the development, progress and sta-
> bility of our respective societies and the world at large and require
> an exceptional and comprehensive global response.[1]

HIV and AIDS have been described as a health issue, a development issue, a
humanitarian issue, and many other issues.[2] Fundamentally, though, HIV
and AIDS remain an issue of justice, rights, and responsibilities, both for those
affected and for those seeking to prevent the spread and mitigate the impact. In
the absence of natural immunity or an effective vaccine, the reality today is that
everyone who is exposed to the virus is susceptible to infection. Exposure to the
virus is most often determined by the risks taken: inadvertently, in ignorance,
by choice, by coercion, or by force. Vulnerability to the risk of infection, and
subsequently to the impacts, is all too often not a straightforward choice and may
be heavily influenced by the prevailing circumstances. Infection with HIV and
the subsequent impact of AIDS have been devastating in the lives of individuals,
families, and communities over the past 30 years.

The church and faith-based organizations (FBOs) have been in the forefront
of response since the earliest days of the epidemic and continue to be amongst the
principle providers of care and support globally. Considerable progress has been
made on the scientific and biomedical front and the advances made in diagnosis
and treatment have changed this disease from a death sentence into a chronically
manageable condition, restoring people living with HIV to active life and once
more giving hope. While such treatment access is being rolled out universally,
there is the disturbing reality that two new infections occur for every one accessing treatment. Not only do new HIV infections continue to outpace response but
the current global financial and economic challenges threaten to undermine the
gains so far achieved. It is increasingly important to constantly reevaluate the way

we do things in order to respond more appropriately, effectively, sustainably, and to an enhanced scale, hence the need to "mainstream" HIV and AIDS. It is an essential process for developing a more inclusive and holistic approach (internally, within the church/FBO sector, and externally, in the responses), which should lead to more effective and comprehensive scale-up, accompanied by both the implementer and especially the primary stakeholders having a sense of ownership.

UNAIDS has suggested that the terminology HIV be used alone and not coupled with AIDS. A person with HIV does not necessarily also have AIDS. HIV is what they are infected with, while AIDS complications is what they die of. The terminology "AIDS" should only be used when specifically referring to AIDS. In this book, however, HIV and AIDS are used together for the specific rational that, while we still have people succumbing to AIDS-related complications, there remains need to be both HIV- *and* AIDS-competent.

Mainstreaming is an evolving process that has been around for some time, but it is a relatively new concept in the area of HIV and AIDS and even more so within the faith community, for which there is limited specific documentation. For a number of years, the World Council of Churches (WCC) has worked on and has been promoting mainstreaming of HIV and AIDS in theological educa-tion. Several accompanying publications have been produced.[3] There are credible initiatives, such as that of the AIDS Constellation promoting the Life Compe-tence Process, and the work of Tearfund (Sue Holden), from which inspiration has been drawn, together with the many life examples and heart-warming initia-tives carried out by churches and faith groups around the world—some of which have been included here as practical examples of what can be done and what is being done.

This handbook seeks to provide guidelines for a possible approach to main-stream HIV and AIDS, as well as guidelines to simultaneously mainstream HIV *competence* into the life and ministry of the church. An HIV- and AIDS-com-petent church denotes a well-informed, inclusive, proactively responsive, and accompanying church. To achieve this involves strong leadership, accurate, up-to-date knowledge, appropriate resources and networks, transforming theology, and compassionate solidarity that restores dignity and hope. To mainstream HIV and AIDS competence is to focus not only on seeking to halt transmission of the virus and to mitigate the impact of infection and of AIDS, but also to focus on those issues that are making people *more vulnerable* to HIV infection and its subsequent impact. It is looking "upstream" at the causes: the socialization process and gender scripting of girls and boys, women and men, that may render each more vulnerable. It involves considering the socioeconomic conditions that promote inequalities, injustices, and poverty, as well as the altered family dynamics and the changing values, fast technology, and media-dominated world in which young people are being raised. It is recognizing the marginalization of minorities and all those considered "different" from ourselves, whereby they are kept in the shadows and are either unable to gain or are denied access to life-giving services. It is challenging the sexual and gender-based violence pervasive in society, where women have little control over their bodies, where girls and women are raped, stigmatized, and made vulnerable to more than HIV alone. It is also recognizing that not only does HIV exist in the church, but also that some people may be made more vulnerable to HIV *because* of working in and for the church and that some of our activities may inadvertently *increase* risks for those we seek to serve.

Mainstreaming also means reviewing critically what actions and activities are currently being undertaken and what needs to be done: looking downstream to mitigate the impact of AIDS.

By mainstreaming HIV and AIDS competence the church can ensure that we do not miss any opportunity to make a significant difference in the lives of individuals, families, communities, and society as a whole. It is "being church." This has been affirmed by Archbishop Anastasios of Tirana and Durres, Orthodox primate of Albania and a WCC President:

> The Mission of the church, and every living member of it, means the obligation and the necessity to share the gifts which we have each received from God. This means to proclaim the truth, love and power revealed by Christ, the crucified and the resurrected one. To share with all everywhere, by the power of the Holy Spirit, with our presence, silence, speech, our acts of love, the fullness of life, the longing for justice and peace all over the world.[4]

HIV has been and remains *a kairos* moment for the church: to be church to humanity and to bring transforming love, health, healing, and restoration of hope and dignity to each and every one, regardless of HIV serostatus, colour, culture, creed, ethnicity, or sexual orientation, for all human life is created in the image of God, is sacred, and is worthy of that promised "abundant life" (John 10:10).

This handbook is divided into ten sections:

- Sections 1 and 2 outline the background to the document, objectives, intended users, and the current scope of HIV and AIDS.
- Section 3 examines why the church should be involved in mainstreaming HIV and AIDS issues and explores the question: "Who is the church?"

- Section 4 discusses what HIV "competence" represents and how this is a fundamental prerequisite to effective mainstreaming.
- Section 5 introduces mainstreaming from a faith perspective where the individual, and the dignity of the individual, is paramount and competence is at the core. The principles, practices, and processes of mainstreaming are described and the distinctions between the internal and external domains of mainstreaming are explored. The *internal domain* represents the internal life and relationships of the church, the "workplace," with the church as an employer, and the recognition that all those who work for and with the church (the "staff")[5] also face risks and vulnerabilities to HIV and impacts of AIDS. The process requires identifying and responding to those factors that are likely to increase vulnerability of church staff and their families to HIV infection. Further engagement requires working to preempt, reduce, or mitigate any possible impacts on the same people. The *external domain* represents the area where the church undertakes activities based on its mandate and core business. Such action is defined by its knowledge of the local context and its available capabilities. Engaging in the external domain requires identifying and then responding to any factors that are likely to increase vulnerability to HIV infection of the individuals and communities with whom the church works and serves. It also involves identifying and reducing possible impacts of HIV and AIDS on these same communities.
- Section 6 introduces the concept of mainstreaming HIV and AIDS into theological institutions.
- Section 7 is devoted to the importance of equipping and journeying with leadership in the understanding and acceptance of HIV, the determinants to its spread, and the magnitude of the impact. Inner transformation is a prerequisite to empowering any technical capacities that may subsequently be developed in order to respond adequately and appropriately.
- Section 8 outlines the process of mainstreaming HIV and HIV competence into specific areas of the church and its various ministries. These include the liturgy, sermons, and homilies, as well as faith formation and moral education in Sunday schools, confirmation classes, and many other associations within the church such as men's, women's, and youth groups, engagement and marriage encounter groups, and various support groups. This section also looks at several programmes that are specifically focused on HIV activities and, in addition, considers the value of ecumenism and interfaith cooperation.

- Sections 9 and 10 are reminders of the necessity of stewardship of time, finances, and resources and the importance of monitoring, evaluation, and information sharing.
- The conclusion completes the document.

The whole document is underscored by three vital issues:

1. The importance of understanding the local context, not only in terms of the specific risks and vulnerabilities present, but also in terms of availability of strategic and important capacities, resources, and services.

2. The value of the appropriate involvement of church staff, congregants, and community, particularly those living with HIV, in a nonjudgmental and respectful manner in the development and implementation of appropriate policy documents and plans.

3. Since no one sector, institution, or individual can address all the aspects of the epidemic, there is need to develop and foster strategic partnerships.[6] Mainstreaming does not require that all components of a comprehensive response to HIV and AIDS be included; however, mainstreaming HIV in the church does require a rational and contextual approach. Activities must be determined on the basis of (a) identified strengths and priority needs, (b) the *comparative advantage* of the church to respond, and (c) its *human and technical capacity* to implement. This may require functional partnerships, networks, and alliances to be formed for appropriate and sustainable implementation and impact.

It should also be remembered that communities do not need to be given dignity, power, or authority; they already have those, though they may need reaffirmation. In all circumstances, there is need to recognize the strengths that are already present in communities, the dreams they have, and their resilience and inherent coping capacities. Sometimes communities are unaware of these strengths, as most programmes are "needs"-focused, and too often focused on *perceived* needs, so that communities become recipients of our solutions rather than being supported, affirmed, accompanied, facilitated, and trained where necessary to find their own solutions. Too often communities have been made to feel that they are victims of their circumstances and that they need to be beneficiaries of our expertise, without which they are unlikely to be capable of any degree of success. They are our partners and resources, not our targets.

> The HIV and AIDS epidemic has taught humanity, perhaps more than anything else before, that a threat to one is a threat to us all: rich and poor, gay and straights, black and white. Let's keep up the good fight. . . . we are one another's neighbour.[7]

Faith-based groups are to be found everywhere, from highly urbanized settings to the most remote rural village. Mainstreaming HIV and AIDS competence is possible in all these settings, and this handbook seeks to outline principles to be followed. Within each local setting, the context may differ, hence the importance of actively engaging with locals to identify priority issues faced within their context: risks, vulnerabilities, availability of alternative choices, back-up services, and specific strengths or needs. The principles remain the same, whatever the context.

> I am come that they might have life, and life *more* abundantly.
> —*John 10:10, KJV*

ACKNOWLEDGMENTS

Beacons of Hope: HIV Competent Churches—A Framework for Action was printed and released in 2008. The book promotes the principles of HIV competence, principally for churches. Considerable interest was shown and the book has been used widely across the globe. Requests started to come on a regular basis on how to turn the principles it expresses into practice. At the same time, the need to mainstream HIV has become more evident. This book has been a "work in progress" ever since and has been presented at various meetings, conferences, and workshops over time. I am extremely grateful to the many people, religious leaders, academics, laypeople, people living with HIV, faith-based organizations, and others, from all over the world, who have contributed ideas, stimulating the thought process, and have generously shared of their experiences.

Grateful thanks go to the many people who have read the different sections and contributed valuable editing advice and ideas, in particular Michael West, Prof. Ezra Chitando, Ben Purcell Gilpin, Ricardo Walters, Lyn Van Rooyen, Fr. Robert Igo, Dr. Manoj Kurian, Calle Almedal, Rev. Dr. Nyambura Njoroge, Rev. Dr. Veikko Munika; Rev. Nelis du Toit, Talitha Rooney, members of the AIDS Constellation process, and many others. Special thanks to Stephanie Purcell Gilpin for help in the design of the diagrammes to accompany the text. Finally, I am indebted to the many organizations and churches who have provided examples of their experiences and programmes, many of which have been included within the text as living examples.

While every effort has been made to identify, contact, and appropriately acknowledge quotations, definitions, and sources of information, any omission is unintentional and sincerely regretted.

Section 1
Why This Handbook?

The World Council of Churches (WCC) has been actively engaged in HIV and AIDS issues since early 1986. In 2002, it established the Ecumenical HIV and AIDS Initiative in Africa (EHAIA) to accompany churches in Africa to respond more effectively and appropriately to HIV and AIDS. This would involve building the capacity of church leadership to eradicate stigma and discrimination through knowledgeable and critical understanding and skills to address the key drivers of the epidemic. It was to be backed up by a transformational life-giving theology that would ultimately create the "AIDS-Competent Church."

1.1 Background

Since 2002 an HIV and AIDS curriculum has been developed and implemented for religious leaders in formation, working in theological institutions, colleges, and universities. Concurrently, extensive training on HIV and AIDS issues has taken place across the continent for religious leaders already in service. This has continued, and expanded, beyond the borders of Africa.

The necessity to mainstream HIV and AIDS into the life and ministry of the church was identified early on and a number of efforts were made in this direction, both by the WCC and by other faith-based organizations and churches. Resource materials have been developed and many consultations have been held in Africa, Southeast Asia, and elsewhere in the world.

In 2008 a WCC-EHAIA resource book entitled *Beacons of Hope: HIV Competent Churches—A Framework for Action* was developed to explore *the principles* of HIV competence for the churches. As the necessity to create HIV-competent churches has become a growing challenge and reality, the need for accompanying guidance on the *practice* of *how to* mainstream HIV competence into the life and ministry of the church became very evident. Hence, this current handbook has been developed as a follow-up to the first book. It seeks to explore what mainstreaming HIV means, especially for the church, determine what the practice of

1

mainstreaming involves, and suggest ways to actually implement the process into
the life and ministry of the church. It is based on experiences and lessons learned
in this field from numerous agencies, faith-based organizations, nongovernmental
organizations, and from WCC-EHAIA. It is complemented by examples of various good practices existing in churches all over the world but principally from
Africa, which has borne the brunt of the epidemic and has suffered greatly from
the impact of AIDS over many years. Included in the document are "checklists"
or "benchmarks" to ease understanding and to act as reference points.

HIV is a dynamic, fast-moving epidemic, and the responses to it change with
the evolving knowledge, experiences, and emerging treatment options. Mainstreaming, too, is an evolving process, not a one-off event, and it is in the same
light that this handbook should be viewed. It remains a work in progress, to be
complemented by the many experiences of the reader and of events still to come.
We are all on a journey.

1.2 Objectives of This Handbook

These are summarized as follows:

- To provide information on approaches to and the importance of mainstreaming HIV into the life of the church;
- To provide practical information on "how to do it" or to strengthen what
has already started (*when, what, why, where, who, and how*);
- To describe how mainstreaming HIV competence into the life of the church
is an extension of the HIV Competence Process that is based on *inner competence, outer competence*, and the bridge between the two of *leadership,
knowledge, and resources*.[1]

1.3 Intended Users

- Leadership of religious institutions and faith-based organizations (FBOs)
- HIV and AIDS focal persons, programme and project staff
- Member churches
- Partners of churches, religious institutions, and FBOs
- Congregants
- Others

The Scope of the HIV and AIDS Epidemic Today

In 2011, world leaders gathered at the United Nations for a General Assembly High Level Meeting on AIDS to restate their commitment to ending the HIV and AIDS epidemic worldwide. In the Political Declaration, they stated: "HIV and AIDS constitute a global emergency, pose one of the most formidable challenges to the development, progress and stability of our respective societies and the world at large and require an exceptional and comprehensive global response."[1] Michel Sidibé, head of the UNAIDS Programme, in 2012 stated, "It has been 30 years since the first reported cases, 15 years since treatment became a reality, 10 years since the first UN General Assembly Special Session on HIV/AIDS and five years since the commitment to achieve universal access to HIV prevention, treatment, care and support."[2]

The vision for the future is: zero new HIV infections, zero discrimination, and zero AIDS-related deaths; to which I believe we should add a fourth goal: that of zero tolerance for sexual gender-based violence.

2.1 The State of the HIV Epidemic[3]

By the end of 2011, 34.2 million people, including 3.4 million children less than 15 years of age, were living with HIV. During the previous 30 years, almost as many (25 million) died of AIDS. This rapidly, relentlessly expanding global epidemic was, by 2006, claiming the lives of more than 2.2 million people each year.

The "revolution" in HIV treatment, resulting from combination anti-retroviral (ARV) therapy released in 1996, forever altered the course of the disease for those living with HIV in high-income countries. It had little impact on low- and middle-income countries, where treatment only reached a fraction of people in need. It is these regions that bear the brunt (90 percent) of the global HIV burden. Significantly, 22 million of the global total of 34 million living in sub-Saharan Africa.

Activists, community leaders, scientists, and health-care providers increasingly demanded access to treatment for all those in need, as well as closure of the gap in health access between the North and the South. Such pressure eventually resulted in increased political and financial commitments to the HIV response, demonstrated in Millennium Development Goals, UN General Assembly Special Sessions on HIV and AIDS, and the creation of funding mechanisms such as the Global Fund, PEPFAR, and UNITAID. These events paralleled the strategic scientific and technical innovations taking place, and so the "impossible" began to look "possible."

A fundamental shift in thinking took place about the feasibility of funding and delivering anti-retroviral (ARV) and other drugs for people in resource-constrained settings. The ensuing rapid scale-up of ARV therapy to eight million people in low- and middle-income countries resulted in a dramatic and significant reduction in the number of people dying from AIDS-related causes, from 2.2 million to 1.8 million per year. Fifty-seven percent of HIV-positive pregnant women received effective therapy to prevent mother-to-child infection. Globally, the annual rate of new infections dropped by 26 percent and the incidence declined in several countries.

The AIDS response saw remarkable progress in 2011, so much so that it has been described as "a game-changing year."[4] The UNAIDS vision of "getting to zero—zero new infections, zero discrimination, and zero AIDS-related deaths" has been embraced by countries, partners, and people around the world, who are working to make it a reality. All UN member states have endorsed the goal of achieving universal access with a package of HIV prevention, care, treatment, and support interventions for all who need them. Former U.S. President George W. Bush stated at ICASA 2011: "We are breaking the grip of AIDS—but this is only the beginning. There is a lot of work to be done. There is no greater priority than saving a human life."

At the 19th International AIDS Conference in Washington, DC, in July 2012, considerable optimism was expressed at the remarkable scientific progress made in the past years, and, for the first time, prominent leaders were beginning to talk about "turning the tide of the HIV epidemic" and the beginning of the end of AIDS, and moving toward "an AIDS-free generation." This would not imply an HIV-free generation, for a cure is yet to be developed. It would mean that no child anywhere would be born with HIV; there would be a significant reduction in the chances of HIV transmission through combination prevention strategies integrating behavioural prevention with biomedical interventions; and for those infected, universal access to sustainable and affordable treatment, care, and support.

Challenges

In spite of the extraordinary achievements, the fresh optimism is also clouded by harsh realities, of which funding is only one. Many challenges remain:

- There are stark regional variations in the HIV seroprevalence and in the responses to the challenge of HIV and AIDS. The seroprevalence in Eastern Europe and Central Asia is noted to be rising again, where the primary mode of transmission is among injecting drug users and their sexual networks, and where deaths from AIDS-related causes increased by 1,100 percent in the past ten years. The annual number of people newly infected with HIV is currently also rising in the Middle East and North Africa.

- Globally, for every person starting ARV therapy, two additional people are infected with HIV. The rate of new infections still outpaces the response.

- Only ten low- and middle-income countries are currently achieving universal targets for ARV therapy.

- The majority of people living with HIV in middle- and low-income countries still do not know their serostatus and hence are not accessing appropriate care and treatment.

- Still less that 50 percent of people in need of ARV treatment are accessing it. Some 30 million will need treatment by 2030 and without significant progress, there will be millions more who are infected in the interim who also in time will require treatment.

- Fewer than one-quarter of children in need of treatment are actually accessing therapy—substantially fewer than adults—a serious situation and justice issue.

- Some 20 percent of people who start on treatment fail to continue and may be lost to follow-up, thus putting themselves at risk and increasing the possibility of developing drug resistance.

- Women are disproportionately affected, especially in Sub-Saharan Africa, principally because of gender inequity and several culturally perpetuated gender norms that increase risk and vulnerability to young girls and women.

- Key populations at higher risk of HIV infection and transmission—injecting drug users, men who have sex with men, transgender people, sex workers, prisoners, and migrants—remain marginalized, face violence, social stigma, and poor access to HIV services. Criminalization in some countries further drives them "underground" and away from care and support.

- Finances: "At a time when mounting evidence indicates that political and financial commitments in the first decade of the 21st century are paying enormous dividends, concerns are growing about the sustainability of the response, the continued upward trajectory of costs and the millions of people in need."[5] "It does not matter how many people can access treatment if we cannot keep them alive and receiving treatment."[6]

- Sharing the burden: There is pressing need for countries to share the responsibility for the global response and take more financial ownership of national AIDS responses by increasing domestic investment in HIV. "Sharing the burden, however, is more than investment—it means collectively tackling the political, institutional, and structural barriers that impede progress. It means ensuring that resources are going where they can have the greatest impact."[7]

New scientific evidence and innovations have continued to expand the tools to deliver on goals. Vaccine research and development continues, with the aim of complete prevention. The scientific community is actively engaged in exploring approaches that may lead to an eventual cure for those already infected. However, we cannot treat our way out of this epidemic and, as UNAIDS concludes in its 2011 Global Report, "innovation goes well beyond scientific discoveries. It is also vital to improve and to bring to scale existing technologies while designing new approaches that can best leverage available resources and optimize outcomes."[8]

As then-U.S. Secretary of State Hillary Clinton stated at the IAS Conference: "This is a fight we can win. We have gone too far to stop now. The USA has made it a priority and we will not back off from achieving this goal."[9]

We know what to do, we know what works, we know the impact of good visionary leadership and the strengths of relevant partnerships, the value of committed advocacy, and the difference that a sensitized, knowledgeable, enabling, and stigma-free environment can make for the lives of all those affected by HIV. If we *want* to make the difference, we can.

In essence, this is what this handbook is seeking to address. It is not about "doing different things, but it is about doing things differently." We want to do the best we can, to the highest standard, in the most relevant and effective ways possible, with maximum use of our resources, time, and effort, reaching both inwards and outwards, and to make a significant, life-affirming difference in the process. In this case, it is about mainstreaming HIV and AIDS issues into the life and ministry of the church; and more, it is about mainstreaming HIV and AIDS *competence* in what we do.

2.2 Determinants of the HIV Epidemic

HIV is no longer seen in terms of being just another medical condition but as an epidemic within other social epidemics of injustice and as a major developmental crisis. It is a disease that affects every aspect of our cultural, spiritual, economic, political, social, and psychological lives.[10]

In countries with a generalized HIV epidemic (where more than 1 percent of the total population is infected), the dominant mode of transmission is through heterosexual sex. In this environment the range of underlying vulnerabilities, in combination, become drivers of HIV infection as well as have an impact on the length and quality of life of those infected and their families. As is evidenced, young women are especially susceptible to HIV infection and vulnerable to the wide-reaching impacts of HIV infection.

Risk factors that are key drivers to the epidemic include:

A. *Structural and social factors*: Individual behaviour is profoundly influenced by the degree to which individuals have financial stability, social control, order, and social cohesion, as well as by the broader contextual factors such as social norms, service accessibility, and public policy. These factors have a considerable influence over their ability and their choices in situations that may present risks of HIV infection. Generally, unequal power relationships; peer pressures; disparity in access to services; physical, cultural, and language barriers; lack of education and employment opportunities; social isolation from familiar support networks (as experienced by migrants, migrant workers, foreigners, truck drivers, displaced persons, and even students) increase vulnerability and affect the choices people make that may put them at risk of HIV infection. Discrimination, inequalities, lower educational status, economic dependence on men, and formidably defended cultural and social norms make it difficult for disempowered women to refuse sex or negotiate for safer sex.

B. *Political factors*: These include governance challenges and the wider implications of national access to (international) resources and services. Access to services may be restricted or barred based on political affiliations and complicated by lack of an enabling environment in which to provide services and support. Conflicts generate and entrench many of the conditions and human rights abuses in which the HIV epidemic flourishes. Conflicts are closely associated with physical and sexual violence, forced displacements and separation from family members, sudden destitution, collapse of social structures, and increased poverty and powerlessness.[11] In addition to the physical and psychological trauma that rape causes, it can also create a cycle of rejection for the victim within her own family and community. All of these challenges can affect delivery of effective HIV services and, again, these invariably have a more severe impact on women.[12]

C. *Biological factors*:
- Gender: Biological, behavioural, and social factors contribute to the increased vulnerability of women—particularly young women—to HIV infection. Anatomically, they are more susceptible to HIV infection, par-

ticularly younger girls with more immature vaginal tracts. Hence, HIV has been described as a feminized epidemic with the numbers of women infected exceeding the numbers of infected men.

- Age: The risk is higher among younger women. The peak of seroprevalence for women is between the ages of 25 and 30, but for men, it is between the ages of 30 and 40.
- Concurrent infections: The risk of HIV infection is substantially increased in the presence of a concurrent sexually transmitted infection.
- Circumcision: Voluntary medical male circumcision offers a partial reduction in HIV risk (68 percent) that, once performed, is lifelong. It does not do away with the need for protected sex in a risky environment, and there is a latent danger in the misconception that circumcision affords complete protection against HIV infection, thus doing away with the need for protection strategies such as condoms.

D. *Behavioural factors*:

- Choice of partners: Whether in a heterosexual or homosexual relationship; whether monogamous and faithful with both partners being aware of their HIV status; or whether in multiple concurrent relationships.
- Choices of sexual practices: Both particular sexual acts and whether or not protection strategies, such as condoms, are used.
- Substance abuse: Excessive alcohol or illicit drug use, particularly injecting drugs and possible use of unsterile needles and syringes.
- Gender formation: The "gender scripting" with which people have been raised that may render them more vulnerable to HIV infection. For instance, in many places, girls are raised to be subservient and submissive to men. They are often left without control over sexual choices. Boys are raised as the machos of society, encouraged to be dominant in relationships and sexual decisions. To have multiple relations is a sign of manhood and power. Both sexes are thus made more vulnerable in an era of HIV.
- The head versus the heart: There is also duplicity in human nature, especially when it comes to sex, between what is known and what is done. There is tension between head knowledge and the "desires of the flesh," and the danger of throwing caution to the wind when the lights go out. The bottom line is that HIV is predominantly transmitted through sex and this is an area we fail to adequately address in our churches.

E. *Gender-based violence (GBV)*: This refers to a range of harmful customs and behaviours against girls and women, including intimate partner violence, domestic violence, assaults against women, child sexual abuse, and rape. It generally derives from cultural and social norms that imbue men with power and authority over women.[13]

GBV can include physical, sexual, and psychological abuse. It is a serious risk factor, which must be acknowledged and addressed if prevention strategies are to have any meaningful effect. Both men and women are exposed to forms of gender-based violence, depending on the circumstances and context in which they find themselves. Increasing evidence connects the expanding HIV epidemic with gender-based violence, particularly among young women.[14]

There should be zero tolerance for abuse of any person or child—whether it occurs in the home, in institutions, on the streets, in the church, in schools, in police stations, in prisons, in refugee centres, or in the area of conflict/war. Regrettably, such abuse often extends to little children, seen as a means of "cleansing" an infected man by sex with a virgin child; this criminal practice is of particular concern.

F. *Negative cultural practices*: Insufficient attention is paid to cultural fundamentals that script women's and men's sexual roles and thus their behaviour patterns. There are also negative cultural practices that increase vulnerability to HIV infection such as: underage marriages, female genital mutilation, unhygienic male circumcision, wife inheritance and widow-cleansing practices, and polygamy coupled with unfaithfulness. Many African Independent Churches, syncretic and traditional religions, which command large adherence, do not have a clear stand on these cultural practices, which are still widely practiced and which can expose people to infection risk.

G. *Economic risks*: These include poverty challenges and insecurity in food, health access and services, housing, and vital transport access. Poverty influences the choices people make, particularly in the case of women resorting to transactional sex work, where HIV risks are manifest, for survival. It may also be connected to behaviour that increases risk of HIV infection such as alcohol abuse, multiple sex partners, and sex for money. Though poor people may not be more at risk to HIV infection than others because of their poverty, it is also true to say that poverty may be coupled with poor underlying nutrition, food insecurity, unsanitary conditions, and unaffordable basic education and health services. HIV is more easily transmitted in these settings. The impact of HIV is most felt at the household level and probably most noted in the area of food insecurity.[15] Widespread movement and migration of people can occur as a consequence of economic pressure, employment availability, climate change, conflicts, and natural disasters. Subsequent isolation from traditional culture and social networks frequently results in risky behaviour.

2.3 Risk, Vulnerability, Susceptibility, and Impact

Throughout the following chapters, there will be reference to risk, vulnerability, susceptibility, and impact. For the purpose of this book, the meanings of these words are explained as follows:

Risk

Risk is the chance taken on an action or activity that potentially could have a negative or harmful outcome. In most instances, taking this chance is a free choice but may be accompanied by ignorance of the likelihood of a negative outcome or the significance of the consequences. It may also be taken under undue pressure or impaired cognitive functions (such as under the influence of alcohol or drugs). In other situations the choice to take the risk is influenced by greater negative circumstances such as, in particular, poverty (which may severely limit freedom of choice), threats of abuse, inability to protect oneself, and cultural practices and beliefs. There are also situations of risk where the person affected does not have any control such as rape, in which there is the possibility of becoming infected with HIV.

Risk is objective. It is not dependent on who you are as a person but what choices you make. It depends on your freedom and ability to make decisions, especially sexual decisions.

Most-affected populations (previously referred to as "most-at-risk populations") have generally tended to be sex workers; sexual minorities, including men who have sex with men; injecting drug users (IDU); prisoners; migrants and mobile populations; truckers; refugees; and internally displaced populations (IDPs). They tend to have a higher prevalence of HIV infection than do the general population, because (a) they engage in behaviors that put them at higher risk of becoming infected and (b) they are among the most marginalized and discriminated-against populations in society.[16]

Vulnerability

Vulnerability is more subjective. It takes "risk" a step further and examines "how" and "why" some groups of people are exposed to much higher levels of risk in their lives. It is the multidimensional situations (biological, social, economic, political, and environmental) that individuals, or communities, experience that may enhance the probability of their being affected by an undesirable outcome. In the case of HIV, vulnerability is a measure of how much control people have over themselves and their sexual health and the risks they take or to which they are exposed. For instance:

- Women whose sexual lives are totally controlled their partners, who may be abusive and unfaithful, are more vulnerable to the risk of HIV infection.
- The physical trauma caused to a child who is raped renders that child more vulnerable to HIV infection.

Vulnerability also implies the likelihood of HIV having collateral negative impacts, for instance, poor households supporting ill relatives are driven into deeper poverty as the costs of care and treatment may consume all available resources and assets.

Susceptibility

Susceptibility is the fact of being exposed. In the absence of a vaccine or natural immunity, everyone is susceptible to HIV infection if exposed to the virus. You can be susceptible but not necessarily vulnerable. For instance:

- Use of a condom reduces susceptibility to infection.
- The poorer you are, the more predisposed or susceptible you are to suffer problems when negative events occur.

Impact

Impact represents the long-term consequences of HIV and AIDS on an individual, family, community, or society. The presence of HIV inevitably results in profound effects in the lives of those infected and affected. For the individual, these range from the physical, emotional, psychological, and economic aspects. At a family level, the presence of HIV in a household may consume all financial resources for health-care expenses; children may be withdrawn from school to care for ailing parents or to act as domestic charges of younger siblings (thus increasing their long-term vulnerability to HIV). Lack of physical manpower and financial resources may increase food insecurity. Orphanhood creates many other challenging dynamics. Timely interventions at the household level with access to effective treatment regimes may result in completely different outcomes and significantly altered impacts.

Even greater impacts may have significance for society as a whole, such as shifts in traditions and societal structure and cultural practices—both positive and negative. Examples include the abandonment of widow-cleansing practices, wife inheritance, and the sex-with-a-virgin myth. On a national level, macroeconomic performance and social policies are also likely to be affected where the epidemic is severe.

2.4 The Need for Mainstreaming HIV and AIDS Competence

It is not knowledge alone that will bring about change. It is not care alone that will ease the plight. A comprehensive response integrating prevention, care, support, and treatment for the HIV-infected and affected is needed within the social reality of the communities we serve. At the same time, we must seek to improve the social and economic circumstances of all, breaking down stigma and challenging injustices. Investment in stigma elimination creates a ripple effect involving whole communities. Recognizing that HIV exists within the church and within the faith community breaks down the barriers and destroys an attitude of "us" and "them." We are all affected in one way or another. By mainstreaming HIV and AIDS into the life and ministry of the church, responding to HIV becomes everyone's business. The battle against HIV will not be won in conference halls, but in homes and communities.

A complete state of competence is not a place we will ever reach. It implies, rather, being on a journey, where we are in progress toward where we want to be. In this, it has the eschatological character of Christian hope.

Why the Church Should Be Involved in Mainstreaming HIV

If your church does not address HIV and AIDS, your ministry is of little relevance in Africa today. —*Evangelical conference speaker, 2008*

Why should the church become involved?

- Because people living with HIV are in churches.
- Because HIV is hurting people and by destroying relationships it is dividing families and communities. HIV is creating generations of hugely disadvantaged orphans and children, whose lives and opportunities are severely compromised due to the insidious and overt impact of HIV on households' ability to cope and the loss of the love and care of the most significant primary carers in their lives.
- Because the church has a comparative advantage to secular interventions.
- Because the church is already involved in development and humanitarian programmes and the linkage between HIV and AIDS and development gaps is well recognized.
- Because the church has a mandate: "Whatever you do to the least of these my brethren, you do to me."
- Because we are not islands. If we are not ourselves directly affected, we certainly all are indirectly affected: "If one part of the body suffers, the whole body suffers."
- Because we can!

HIV and AIDS have disturbed our comfort zone and our conventional theologies have been challenged, making us face our inadequacies and our prejudices in the light of the Lord's transforming love. It has been and remains a *kairos* moment for the church, to *be* church to humanity and to bring transforming love, health, healing, and restoration of hope and dignity to each and every one, regardless of HIV status, colour, culture, creed, ethnicity, or sexual orientation. For all human life is created in the image of God and is sacred and is worthy of that promised "abundant life."

3.1 The Comparative Advantage of the Church

> In the Church and Faith Based Organisations, there is great potential to be prophets, healers, and reconcilers. It is vital that more attention is given to increasing the competency of Church leaders and to building the capacity for all organisations working and ministering with HIV and AIDS.
> —*Message from the Pre-Assembly of People Living with HIV to the 13th General Assembly of the Christian Conference of Asia, 17 April 2010*[1]

There are many actors in the response to HIV and AIDS. What makes the church different?

Churches complement governments and other agencies in their service provision but churches tend to reach out to the poorest of the poor and provide services where no one else goes. There is more, however; churches own and are extensively involved in the provision of medical services, through their hospitals, clinics, mobile units, and home-based care; and in the provision of education through their schools, colleges, universities, training centres, and theological institutions. Churches are also extensively involved in humanitarian and developmental services, as well as gender programmes and a multitude of other outreaches. They have physical structures and are packed with volunteers from all walks of life and professions. They have, in fact, the largest constituency, stretching from the most remote village to the international community. Because of their continued presence in the communities and their engagement with people during the most significant times of life (birth, marriage, illness, death), they have an earned credibility and trust and, what is more, they have a "higher mandate," not simply a "calling."

The church is there for the long haul. It does not come and go with elections or when the going gets tough. Long after all the secular agencies have left, in the midst of conflict and other crisis, the church is still there. It is our mandate. As such, we do not speak of "an exit strategy" from the people. The church is there to support, empower, accompany, advocate for social justice, and be in solidarity with all those in need. It asks for no reward save that of doing the will of God and serving God's people. Thus, in all the HIV and AIDS programmes, the church seeks to walk alongside the communities as they respond to their challenges and rise above the impacts. The church seeks to eliminate stigma and discrimination, to restore dignity, and to offer solace and compassion for those whose hope has been dimmed. The church is there as a beacon of hope and a conduit for God's unconditional love for God's people. Therein lies our difference in our response to HIV and to any other issue that presents a life-threatening challenge to the people of God.

If churches can mainstream HIV competence in the institution of the church, in Christian educational systems, in church health institutions, and into all other services, they potentially have the greatest reach of any sector. They could have, by far, the largest impact on raising awareness, counteracting stigma, exposing injustices and inequalities, engaging in advocacy, empowering people to halt the transmission of the virus, and effectively mitigating its impact.

To achieve such an end requires committed, motivated, and motivating leadership with sound knowledge, as well as good and strong partnerships all supported with appropriate and adequate resources. By mainstreaming HIV competence into the life and ministry of the church, HIV response becomes part of the core business of the church, not merely an add-on.

3.2 The Church's Current Response

For some 30 years, we have been faced with a growing HIV epidemic, an epidemic that continues to outpace responses despite all the improved understanding of the virus and the major medical advances available to control its effects. Each and every day, 4,900 people die of AIDS-related conditions while 7,100 new HIV infections occur.[2] Alarmingly, at the very heart of our society, young people, girls, and women continue to be the most affected group.

It is well acknowledged that faith-based organizations (FBOs) play a substantive and critical role in the provision of health services and care rights across Africa, representing between 30 and 70 percent of all care that is provided.[3] While parishes and congregations have, since the onset of the epidemic, been in the forefront of care and support initiatives, their level of response, and the quality and coverage, is in no way commensurate with the size of this growing epidemic. In spite of evidence that empowering people slows the spread of the virus, the many efforts to mitigate its impact on individuals, families, and communities, though commendable, are still not halting the tide. If we as the church are serious about making a genuine difference, then it is not right that we rely on the hard work and efforts of the few amongst us who serve so faithfully. HIV is and must become everyone's business in the church. It affects us all now and certainly will continue to affect us more and more, if we do not make it so.

> The very relevance of the church will be determined by their response. The crisis also challenges the churches to re-examine the human conditions, which in fact promote the pandemic, and to sharpen their awareness of people's inhumanity to one another, of broken relationships and unjust structures, and their own complacency and complicity. HIV and AIDS is a sign of the times, calling us to see and to understand. —*World Council of Churches*[4]

> If the church does not take care of AIDS, AIDS will take care of the church. —*Anonymous*

It can no longer be "business as usual." We need to rethink the way we are doing things, the way we understand the virus, our acceptance that HIV and AIDS are right in our midst, and that perhaps our responses, as noble as they are, are in fact missing essential targets. Who is at risk? Why are there risks? Is there clear understanding of the risks? What should we do about them? What is making people vulnerable to HIV and its impacts? Further, are we in fact contributing to the problem rather than effectively addressing it, either through silence, inaction, or misguided action?

By mainstreaming HIV and AIDS competence into the life and ministry of the xhurch, we effectively view all that we do and seek to do through "wearing AIDS glasses."

3.3 Who Is "The Church"?

> We are Christians, not because we believe in God, but because of the God we believe in. —*Father Abel Makahamadze, C.Ss.R.*

> In many instances, we tend to assume that "the church" refers to the institutional body that owns buildings and other properties. In this scheme, "the church" is a structure that is "out there." The scheme presents "the church" as an impersonal institution that is concerned with administrative issues and upholding accepted

theological standards. Such an interpretation of the church distances church leaders from lay people. It presents the church hierarchically, with those in authority taken to be (in a sense) an embodiment of the church. This leaves lay people at the bottom of the structure. Power is taken to reside with those who hold leadership positions (the ordained), while lay people are supposed to follow the direction suggested by those in the ordained ministry.

An interpretation of the church that adopts the hierarchical model is deficient. There is need to recognize that "the church" means "the whole body of Christ." The church is not "out there" but is "here now." The church is not the exclusive possession of those who are ordained and have leadership positions. The church is constituted by all believers who regularly participate in its activities and confess its faith. When we say, "the church must . . . ," we are in fact challenging every individual believer to use his or her energy to endeavor to accomplish the set goals and targets. The church does not exist in the abstract—outside the efforts of its members—but exists in the actions of each one of the believers. In this context, "the church" must be understood as the concerted efforts of lay and ordained members working with God to realize the kingdom of God. —*Ezra Chitando*[5]

When we . . . declare, "the Church has done much . . . and much more is needed," we can easily think they mean a more sophisticated response on a larger scale. But as Cardinal Turkson said . . . the Church is the only institution that meets hundreds of people each week on a very personal level and at the same time acts publicly and socially. Who else can do both so regularly? In its AIDS ministry, the Church faces the biggest combined social, cultural, economic, medical and political issues and, at the same time, she deals with individual persons one by one, those infected by [HIV and AIDS] and their family much affected by it. So to say "much more is needed" does not mean "bigger and more complex"; it means multiplying the small-scale, close-to-the-ground, highly personal approaches and extending them to more and more people infected and affected. The response of the Church to [HIV and AIDS] needs to be as extensive, broad and deep as the mission of the Church herself. . . . So let us be clear: [HIV and AIDS], for the Church, is a huge problem, but it is not a "massive" one to be addressed on a large scale and in the millions. Rather, there is and will be a great variety and nearly infinite multiplicity of genuinely pastoral responses. This is how the Church tackles a huge problem like sin, or ignorance, or [HIV and AIDS]. —*Michael Czerny, S.J.*[6]

HIV and AIDS Competence

The most powerful agent of growth and transformation is something more basic than any technique: a change of heart.
—John Welwood

The heart of the matter is a matter of the heart. *—Roy Musasiwa*

The first step for any church or faith-based organization is the need to unpack the risks that HIV poses to ourselves and to our church, in order to be sufficiently convinced and thus motivated to carry mainstreaming further into actual practice, both within the church and in all the many activities and outreaches of the church.

Over time, various stakeholders and organizations working in the field of HIV have developed different definitions of HIV and AIDS competence. In reality it can mean different things to different people and understanding of competence changes with the evolution of the epidemic.

For the churches, the following definition has been developed:

An HIV-competent church is a church that has first developed *an inner competence* through internalization of the risks, impact, and consequences and has accepted the responsibility and imperative to respond appropriately and compassionately. In order to progress to *outer competence*, there is need for *leadership, knowledge, and resources. Outer competence* involves building theological and institutional capacity in a socially relevant, inclusive, sustainable, and collaborative way that reduces the spread of HIV, improves the lives of the infected and affected, mitigates the impact of HIV and ultimately restores hope and dignity.[1]

4.1 Inner Competence

> We need to begin the journey towards ourselves before we begin
> a journey towards the other and towards God.
> —*Justa Paz Organization*[2]

HIV competence, from a faith perspective, brings the challenge home, first and foremost, to ourselves. We are challenged to consider and to reflect on facts, and realities, and to acknowledge and accept that HIV is a condition that can affect and infect *anyone,* including ourselves and those closest to us. It means consideration of sexual behaviours, mindsets, attitudes, and values. It involves challenging our preconceptions and our current responses. It involves facing the reality of stigma, discrimination, and denial. HIV stigma reflects human values, heart issues, and stems from fear, ignorance, anxieties, prejudices, and rigid attitudes. Those who stigmatize often want to be seen as people of high moral standards. These attitudes are to be found within our churches and within ourselves, negating our authenticity and credibility as people of love seeking to serve others.[3] It means relooking at our theologies and challenging negative theologies that are not life giving. It also means recognizing the devastating impact HIV and AIDS has had, is having, and will have on the lives of individuals, families, communities, and on society as a whole. It is thus making a conscious decision to be changed—to be transformed—and to ensure that whatever we do is relevant, based on factual evidence, and done with compassion to restore dignity and hope. This is the path to inner competence.

This is the "heart" of our response and is at the core of any mainstreaming process in our faith settings. Anything and everything else that we do should springboard from such inner transformed convictions.

> Everyone thinks of changing the world, but no one thinks of
> changing himself. —*Leo Tolstoy*

Without an inner transformation on the way *we* understand HIV and AIDS and its potentially devastating impact on individuals, on ourselves, families, communities, and society as a whole, any external HIV activities undertaken may lack authenticity.

> The major challenge is not to focus on what congregations are
> *doing* in terms of HIV and AIDS, but rather to first focus on who
> we *are* as church and how we identify with HIV and AIDS. We

> therefore need to establish a culture of vulnerability and a true
> identification with the HIV positive body of Christ, not because
> we know one or several people who are living with HIV, but
> because we acknowledge that the church is vulnerable and deeply
> affected by HIV. We believe this understanding will fundamen-
> tally change the way this task group supports congregations.
> —*CABSA Network*[4]

Once there is recognition and acceptance that HIV can affect anyone, even within our own ranks, then there is need to look more deeply at these risks and the key drivers of the epidemic that are facilitating the spread of HIV within our communities and within society as a whole.

> We want the facts to fit the preconceptions. When they don't, it is
> easier to ignore the facts than to change the preconceptions.
> —*Jessamyn West*

4.2 Outer Competence[5]

As churches, the effectiveness and relevance of our activities, that is, our outer competence, is directly related to the extent to which we have sought to become theologically and technically competent, socially relevant and inclusive, col-laborative, and advocates for social justice, so that we might truly restore hope and dignity.

Theologically Competent

Theological competence involves honest reflections on our theology in the era of HIV. This involves dealing with questions such as: Is AIDS punishment from God? Where is God in all this suffering? What kind of healing can we hope for in the context of HIV? In addition, the subject of sex and sexuality needs to be unpacked in an open and honest way, breaking the silence and ensuring accurate life giving information is shared. Scripture has often been manipulated to rein-force gender oppression and unequal power relations. The recognition that sex and sexuality is a gift from God has been downgraded and treated as something sinful, debased, lustful, unholy, to be hidden and definitely not celebrated for its inherent beauty and true holistic purpose. Gender relations need to be examined in a life-affirming way.

Technically Competent

Technical competence is developed through finding ways to improve or to build the church's or institution's capacity to plan, implement, monitor, and coordinate HIV programmes effectively. Skills should be developed through participation and learning. Technical competence also requires developing regular systems of follow-up, monitoring, and impact.

Socially Relevant and Inclusive

Social relevance and inclusiveness is about building relationships around what matters and promoting in those relationships a sense of belonging, of feeling respected and valued, and an experience of support and commitment that is encouraging and motivating. This is a process toward building social cohesion, which is society's capacity to ensure the well-being of *all* its members, minimizing disparities and avoiding marginalization.

There are structural sins in society—inequities and inequalities; attitudes and acts that degrade, oppress, or exclude others—that negatively influence the choices people are able to make. These need to be addressed. For example: the difficult and limited choices left to the widow, with low educational status and poor economic prospects because she is a woman, who is deprived of all her material possessions by greedy relatives. Left with nothing to support her children, she may resort to sex work, and plenty of people will be willing to exploit her desperate situation. Yet society will both stigmatize her and accuse her of being responsible for the spread of HIV. HIV is a justice issue and responses should not focus on just giving handouts to the poor but addressing the systems and structures that keep the poor in their misery. Society is full of socially dislocated people, isolated from their usual support systems. The church can play an unrecognized prevention role by being a home, an anchor, a place where there is reinforcement of positive value systems and loving compassionate peer support. It may provide a social network and sense of inclusion and *a safe space.*

> The church can still be the place where believers feel comfortable
> to talk about their HIV status in the confidence that they will
> receive the support that they deserve.
> —*Retired South African Archbishop Desmond Tutu*

We must ensure that all programmes do not discriminate against nor exclude any persons. The process of inclusion should involve each individual in a way that they

feel valued and part of the success of the programme. The meaningful involvement of people living with HIV enriches all programmes as there is so much to learn from their firsthand experiences. People living with HIV are not just "the problem"; they are part of the solution. People long to be treated with respect and dignity in processes that empower as opposed to scenarios that involve coercion.

Collaboration and Networking

Although churches often believe themselves to be self-sufficient and therefore work in isolation, HIV is affecting all our communities and thus there is merit in networking and collaborating with others who are working in similar fields. This enables better coordination, less duplication and gaps, and increased scale and sustainability. It also affords the opportunity for shared experiences and shared resources where appropriate.

Where churches are providing home-based care and local orphan support, such volunteers have a wealth of experience and exposure to the lived realities of the people they visit and support. Such experience could fruitfully inform health clinics, OVC programmers, and policymakers on what works and what is not working. They, too, can be useful conduits of information between secular sectors and the affected individuals, families, households, and communities, as well as play a pivotal role in encouraging testing and treatment adherence, while providing psychosocial support and ongoing accompaniment.

The church also has its own extensive networks through its schools, health facilities and delivery systems, development and humanitarian departments, as well as gender and justice desks. These can be more fully utilized, especially if it is recognized that HIV cuts across all these systems and departments.

Advocacy and Mobilization for Social Justice

> Speak up for those who cannot speak for themselves, for the rights
> of all who are destitute. Speak up and judge fairly; defend the
> rights of the poor and needy. —*Proverbs 31:8-9, NIV*

It is said that advocacy is any attempt to influence public opinion and attitudes that directly affect people's lives. HIV is a human rights and social justice issue. Church leadership must reclaim its prophetic voice to advocate for policies that address social inequalities and help the voiceless regain their voice in the struggle for social reform. Governments should be held accountable to the constitutions and conventions to which they are signatories. At the international and regional level, there is much room for diplomatic and supragovernmental pressure, not just governmental pressure.

Churches can mobilize community coalitions to work for local solutions to the challenges caused by HIV and AIDS. They can help build the capacity of community leaders to facilitate positive change in their communities to significantly improve the lives of those most affected by social injustices.

Compassionate in Restoring Hope and Dignity

The ultimate object is to prevent HIV, mitigate its effects, share good practices, bring relief, and, most of all, accompany those of us who are infected and affected on the journey of HIV. This solidarity and support can help to restore dignity and hope and a valued place in society.

4.3 Bridge of Leadership, Knowledge, and Resources

The bridge between inner and outer competence is achieved through *leadership, knowledge,* and *resources.*

- *Leadership* implies not only hierarchy but all those in positions of influence. All leadership needs to be adequately informed and properly trained to counteract irrational fears and misconceptions about HIV. Leaders need to be accountable and dependable, those who "stay the course." True leaders lead by example, with humility and faithfulness. True leadership does not imply taking or leading people to where they want to go. Sometimes it implies leading people not necessarily to where they *want* to go but to where they *ought* to go. Jesus is our role model, a true leader who chose not to rule but to serve, and who led by the deeply challenging example of the one whose all-encompassing sacrificial love superseded any personal cost in order to bring us to the place of reconciliation with God and with our neighbor.

- *Knowledge (of HIV and AIDS).* It is said that information is one of the most powerful tools available to create positive social change. It may bridge the gap between poverty and opportunity. In the era of HIV and AIDS, it may mean the difference between life and death. Hence it is vitally important for information on HIV and AIDS to be accurate, up-to-date, factual, and relevant, recognizing the determinants of its spread, including social factors, and that this information is shared with and understood by all those who need to know. It also involves being critically aware of the impact of HIV and AIDS on individuals, families, communities, and the church itself.

- *Knowledge (local).* General knowledge on the virus is insufficient if one is seeking to respond appropriately and effectively. It is also vital to also be fully informed on the local situation where one is seeking to serve. Acquisition of such local knowledge may need to be based on assessments carried out to ascertain the extent of HIV in the community and its impact, as well as knowledge of the availability and accessibility of services, including information, prevention, testing and counseling centers, care, support, and treatment. Where do the community members go or where *can* they go for the information and services that they need to deal with HIV in their lives? To whom could they be referred if the church is unable to meet their immediate needs? How do families deal with stress? How do they make their way through life together? This elevates the analysis beyond just the material and clinical needs and service interventions.

- *Resources* mean more than mere financial resources. There are also structural resources, which include church buildings, halls, meeting spaces, schools, and hospitals; human resources and the many skills available; as well as many resource materials, training manuals, toolkits, and multiple links with and to the international community. Our spiritual resources are many.

These three—leadership, knowledge, and resources—need to be rooted in the communities that are being served, reflecting their experiences, challenges, and expressed needs. Meaningful involvement of those who are most affected, coupled with collaboration with other key stakeholders ensures respect and the development of responses that are appropriate and based on the lived reality of the recipients and not on the perceived reality of those who are seeking to respond.

Within the faith context, it is my belief that internal mainstreaming is a logical extension of inner competence, just as external mainstreaming is a logical extension of outer competence. *Inner and outer competence must underpin any mainstreaming efforts.*

By first establishing who we are as church and how we identify with HIV and AIDS, and how we identify with the "HIV-positive body of Christ," we have the opportunity to experience a deeper understanding of the complexities of HIV and to undergo and embrace an inner transformation of ourselves and our attitudes. This is possible both as individuals and as the church or faith institution. Transformation leads to engagement and to proactive action, to make a positive difference in the lives of those amongst us who have been affected by HIV.

Mainstreaming

Mainstreaming is not a new process in the secular world. It is increasingly recommended as a mechanism for tackling HIV and AIDS, gender, and human rights in a more effective and sustainable way. There is no standard way of undertaking it, as the approach is determined usually by the epidemic stage, the specific cultural context, and the challenges and opportunities presented. It is, however, most recognized for its two components: *internal mainstreaming* and *external mainstreaming.*

5.1 Mainstreaming from a Faith Perspective

This handbook looks at more than mainstreaming HIV and AIDS; it looks at mainstreaming HIV and AIDS *competence,* from a faith perspective. As such, it adds another dimension to the discourse and practice, that of *inner and outer competence,* as a prerequisite to effectively and sustainably mainstreaming, both internally and externally.

There is no blueprint on how to mainstream HIV competence in churches. While most other sectors, in addressing mainstreaming HIV and AIDS, have focused on HIV and its impact directly on each particular sector and the beneficiaries, churches are in the unique position to go further and deeper. Thus they can address the issues that tend to remain "under the table" which are at the root of HIV transmission—those things cloaked in silence and that put people at risk and those that increase vulnerability. HIV is an end consequence of a number of factors. It is these factors that need to be acknowledged and addressed if our messages on HIV are to have any meaningful impact in the lives of both the uninfected and the affected.

We cannot, however, respond with real authenticity if we have not first faced our own susceptibility, attitudes, fears, and beliefs. Our attitudes and values are ultimately reflected in our behaviour, skills, and responses.

5.2 The Basics of Mainstreaming

Many commonly accepted comprehensive responses to HIV and AIDS tend to focus on the medical aspects of HIV in terms of transmission, prevention, testing, treatment, care and support, and behavioural responses to HIV, as well as on mitigating the impact. Mainstreaming, however, is a learning process that focuses on addressing the causes and effects of HIV and AIDS and the impacts, in an effective and sustainable way, in the workplace and in the day-to-day work practices.[1]

Integration or Mainstreaming?

These two terms are often thought to mean the same thing. In practice, however, they are not.

Integration occurs when HIV- and AIDS-related issues and interventions are introduced into a project, programme, or policy context as a component or content area, without much interference with the specific core business of the institution or the main purpose of the policy instrument.[2] It basically means *adding on* components that address HIV and AIDS issues.

Mainstreaming, however, is more than integration. It is not implementing HIV and AIDS activities along with or as part of other programmes. It becomes aligned with, and in turn influences, the core business of an institution, thus becoming more than an "add-on." It means understanding how HIV may change the context in which one works and thus affect the nature of the work that is done. It means considering whether or how programmes may reduce or inadvertently increase vulnerability and how specific programmes can respond to vulnerability to HIV and its impacts, given the particular expertise and comparative advantage of the church in this situation.[3] It means "wearing AIDS glasses" while working in all sectors and at all levels.

What Mainstreaming HIV and AIDS Does *Not* Mean[4]

- Pushing HIV into programmes where it is not relevant.
- Changing core functions and responsibilities in order to turn all activities into HIV and AIDS programmes.
- Simply introducing HIV and AIDS awareness in all our activities.
- That we all have to become HIV specialists.
- Business as usual.

"Mainstreaming is about challenging the status quo by looking upstream to see the deep developmental causes and downstream to appreciate the wide impacts of HIV and AIDS."[5] Mainstreaming does not always mean doing something new but it can mean modifying what is already being done to make it more HIV- and AIDS-specific and relevant. It is not necessarily extra work but adds value to the activities.

Mainstreaming has many facets, including, critically, changes in accepted norms, values, and established systems in individuals and in the institutions. It is not a one-off event; it is a continuous process. Both the context and the epidemic itself are dynamic, and so should be the responses.

Key Capacities Needed for Effectively Mainstreaming HIV and AIDS Competence[6]

- Basic knowledge and understanding of HIV and AIDS—determinants to the spread of HIV, the drivers of the epidemic, and the potential impacts; prevention strategies, including treatment options; the basics of care and support; an understanding of the implications of gender inequalities and gender-based violence in relation to HIV; an understanding of the effects of stigma—are essential.
- Understanding how HIV and AIDS are affecting the church, both internally and externally.
- Understanding of the church's response to HIV and the potential for the church to unwittingly enhance vulnerability to HIV infection or undermine existing coping capabilities to deal with the consequences of HIV.
- Skills to apply this knowledge to the everyday functioning of the church and to translate understanding and knowledge into effective and relevant actions.
- Always involving people living with HIV and those personally affected by HIV in all stages of planning, decision making, and, where appropriate, implementation as well.
- Advocating, communicating, transferring learnings, sharing experiences, and motivating others to take a stand on HIV and AIDS.

5.3 Guiding Principles

Mainstreaming is first and foremost about *people*: people who work in the church or organizations and people who are affected by what we do and how we do it. It is not possible to talk of an effective response to HIV without including gender, as it is inextricably linked with HIV.

Mainstreaming has many facets, including a process of individual and institutional change. It is a continuous process requiring commitment to long-term institutional transformation that changes norms, values, and systems to bring about new and comprehensive results. It is best carried out by a team. Strong leadership may be the linchpin that helps to build a consensus around the vision and encourages commitment at every level within the church, its structures, and institutions. It also requires a strong motivating belief that the church can develop the capacity needed, can align with other HIV and AIDS stakeholders, and can ensure effective, accountable, and transparent use of resources.

There are two predominant areas for action: the *internal domain* and the *external domain*.

1. *The internal or workplace domain* focuses on the vulnerabilities and risks of the people who work within or for the church, church institutions, and church projects and programmes. It is here that we question and seek to respond to the way HIV and AIDS are affecting our church and its ability to work effectively, both now and in the future.

2. *The external and target community domain.* HIV is mainstreamed into the core mandate, activities, and business of the church and church-owned facilities or projects. Serving in the communities, it takes into account and reacts to eliminate or reduce susceptibility of community members to HIV infection and vulnerability to the impacts of HIV and AIDS.

Understanding and internalizing HIV issues, changing attitudes and being transformed (inner competence in the internal domain of the church) will have a direct influence on what and how the church responds externally.

The overall goal of mainstreaming HIV competence is to ensure that the church is HIV-knowledgeable, inclusive, compassionate, competent, and relevant in all its responses to HIV and AIDS, and that the dignity and human rights of all who work within or for the church, or those who benefit from the work of the church, are respected and upheld. It is also to ensure that all programmes address both the causes of and the effects of the HIV epidemic, reduce susceptibility to HIV and vulnerability to its impact, and make a positive difference for those living with or personally affected by HIV.

5.4 Internal Mainstreaming HIV and AIDS Competence

"Internal mainstreaming" involves looking *into* the church and the people within the church as employees or workers/staff who are responsible for the running of the church and its programmes. It should involve employees at every stage to help break the silence about HIV and its impacts within the church.

It is a process that involves identifying and responding to factors—individual, organizational, and societal—that are likely to increase vulnerability to HIV infection for church staff, immediate family members, and community. It is also recognizing and preempting, reversing, or mitigating likely impacts of HIV and AIDS on the staff and on the church as a whole.[7]

The church may, in many instances and particularly in the mainline churches, be a significant employer with employees engaged in church administration at all levels, in pastoral care, and within the many institutions run by the church, including the provision of health and education and in development and extension work. It also is packed with volunteers who give freely of their time and skills but nevertheless are "working" within the church.

The church has consistently affirmed the dignity of labour, for example, as in Pope John Paul II's encyclical: ". . . the basis for determining the value of work is not primarily the work being done but the fact that the one doing it is a person."[8] Work is for people, not people for work. Through work, individuals not only transform the world but also achieve fulfillment as human beings.[9] However, there are fundamental principles of morality and social justice that should form the basis of promoting good relationships between the employer (the church) and the employee in the contemporary world. In an environment where HIV and AIDS are a reality in the life of the church and of our communities, it is of the utmost importance to strive to understand the magnitude of the impact of HIV and AIDS, currently, on the staff.

A suggested step-by-step process of mainstreaming HIV and AIDS competence internally in the church (Int. Ms.) is as follows:

Int. Ms. 1: Our Vision

Start with the identification of a vision of what you would like to see and to have in place in the church, for all those who work in and for the church. For example:

> HIV and AIDS competence mainstreamed into the life of the church and all its internal domains, recognizing the prevalent risks and vulnerabilities to HIV and AIDS, and responding appropriately and compassionately to prevent or reduce such risks and vulnerabilities as well as mitigating the impacts of AIDS on the people who work in and for the church.

How can we achieve this? The operative word is "we," as it implies *all* of us and is inclusive. People living with HIV or personally affected should also be involved in the dialogue and planning, as they bring the lived experience to the discussions. Involving key stakeholders from the outset acknowledges the vital role they play in the functioning of the church and creates a sense of ownership to the process.

All stakeholders need to understand the value of mainstreaming competence and be committed to the process through maximizing current strengths and opportunities and addressing the gaps and barriers to achieve the agreed vision. Before any action can be undertaken, however, it is necessary to honestly appraise "Where are we now?" through exploring how HIV and AIDS are affecting the church.

Int. Ms. 2: Where Are We Now?
Int. Ms. 2.1: Undertake an Organizational Analysis

To establish how HIV and AIDS are currently affecting the church requires a thorough and honest appraisal of the situation and the threats that HIV is presenting. In essence, there is need to review how HIV and AIDS are affecting those who work in/for the church, what is putting them at risk and increasing their vulnerability to HIV infection, and how this will affect the functioning of the church, now and in the future.

A. *How are those who work in and for the church affected by HIV and AIDS?* Focus carefully on the people who serve or work in the church, including ourselves, and on those within the varied church-run institutions and programmes, whether in positions of leadership, as mission hospital staff, as teachers in church-owned educational institutions, as general employees in any of the numerous church-run departments, or as volunteers, even the people who tidy the garden or sweep the church. At this stage, this focus does not necessarily include the members of the congregation who *attend* the services of the church, or the people and community who benefit from the activities of the church. Here the focus is on those who work and serve within the domain of the church/faith-based institution, whether as paid employees, those following a vocation, or as volunteers.

B. *Risks.* Consider how those serving in the church are already affected by the reality of HIV. What are the personal experiences of HIV?

- Explore attitudes, beliefs, prejudices, understandings, fears, myths, and misconceptions about HIV infection and about AIDS and its consequences. What do the "employees" know, talk about, and understand about HIV and AIDS and gender-based violence? Take note of language used that may be stigmatizing. Include exploration of attitudes toward people with alternative sexual orientations.
- Explore the depth of knowledge and understanding of HIV: methods of transmission and prevention; window period; signs and symptoms of infection; testing; opportunistic infections; treatment and the necessity for

treatment adherence; effects of stigma; key drivers of the epidemic; gender disparities and violence; and the manifestations of AIDS.

- Do people recognize the risks and see HIV as any form of threat to them personally or to their families?
- Are people in denial about risks? What coping strategies are already in place?
- There will be those who are personally affected by HIV, either actually living with HIV or affected through close association with others who are living with HIV. It is important to sensitively understand how they are coping. What resources or forms of support do they lack and need? How does this situation affect their ability to do their work?
- Develop a demographic and socioeconomic profile of the people who serve the church as a baseline and look at what might be putting people at risk of HIV and increasing their vulnerability to infection. For example, take note of mobility in relation to the work: How frequently and for how long does their work take them away from their nuclear families? Seek to understand the norms and values that are driving the workforce; for instance, power relations, gender disparities, sense of self-worth, alcohol consumption, exposure to violence, and any known risk behaviours.[10]
- Identify common health problems and levels and trends of staff turnover. What percentage might be attributed to HIV infection?

C. *Vulnerability to HIV infection.* How does the working in or for the church increase the vulnerability of the staff and volunteers to HIV infection?

Just as the church may offer protection, advice, and support to those who work for the church, some working situations within the church may increase the vulnerability of these same people to HIV. Consider carefully, together with all whom it may affect, what these working situations may be and, by recognizing the interlinkages between HIV and their work, together plan ways to reduce these risks. For example:

- Health workers might not be provided with protective gloves.
- Priests and pastors may be stationed in remote areas, without emotional and psychological support. Working alone, they are under a lot of stress and face enormous expectations and may become lonely and seek solace from sources that may make them more vulnerable to the risks of HIV.
- The church usually does not pay salaries competitive with the secular world. Low pay or late payments may drive people concerned to seek to supplement their income in ways that render them more at risk to HIV infection. Adoption of risky behaviour increases susceptibility and vulnerability.

- Having women travel alone to the field on pastoral visits, providing home-based care and other caring ministries, may put them in less-than-safe settings. This makes them vulnerable to potential abuse and thus additional risks.
- Power positions and dynamics, particularly when attributed to men, may result in sexual harassment or demands for sex from those in lesser positions of power. Particularly in rural settings, female workers are vulnerable to exploitation and male workers may take unwise risks.
- Lack of care for the caregivers and absence of appropriate coping mechanisms in situations of work overload and excessive stress may increase the vulnerability of the church worker or caregiver to careless risks.

D. *Available policies/instruments/resources.* Explore whether there are already in place policy documents or church instruments that can be called upon or modified appropriately to ensure they take into consideration and are appropriate to the context of HIV and AIDS and its implications.

Int. Ms. 2.2: Impact Assessment

If people who work in the church are both infected and affected by HIV, how will this affect the work of the church and its ability to work effectively now and in the future? The effect is likely to be experienced within the human resources—the people who work in and for the church—in the functioning of the church, and in the financial implications. To measure this impact may require a baseline survey.[11]

A. *Impact on those who work in and for the church.* The impact on the work of the church may be most noticed in increasing levels of sickness, absenteeism, loss of skills, increased work load, and demands on remaining church staff, who may have to multitask, which in turn may lead to high stress levels, fatigue, and being unable to work effectively. The general morale of staff may be affected, not only from the additional workload, but also from the loss of friends and colleagues.

Staff may be under increased financial pressures as a result of health expenses, support for ill family members, or the additional strain of support for extras—such as unemployed ill relatives or care for children orphaned as a consequence of AIDS. They may be under considerable emotional and psychological stress as well, especially if there are limited opportunities for support and encouragement.

B. *Impact on the work of the church.* The loss of key people and skills may mean that the church is unable to do what it had planned; thus sustainability may be affected. Furthermore, efficiency is also affected as documentation may lag behind, coping mechanisms may be eroded, and institutional memory is lost.

The financial impact cannot be overlooked as HIV and AIDS are both costly, in terms of actual funds and in terms of the excessive strain they place on the individual and family assets and resources. For the church there is the cost of sick leave and compassionate leave; finding resources to assist with medical expenses and to support families; and salaries paid but work left undone. In addition, there are the costs of fresh recruitment or overlap employment, the training of new personnel, and the additional time taken in management supervision. Yet the training and recruitment may not be enough to cope with the pressures created by HIV, and systems may not be in place for planning and monitoring and ongoing skills requirements.[12]

The combined data of the baseline survey you conduct should give an indication of the current understanding of the basics of HIV and the current (and possible future) impact of HIV and AIDS on the staff of the church.

Exploring these key questions and issues gives a broader understanding of the reality and of the magnitude of the impact of HIV and AIDS on the internal domain of the church. It provides opportunities to look at current strengths and gaps and to strategize to address risks, reduce vulnerabilities, build the capacity to cope, and mitigate against these impacts.

Int. Ms. 3: What Do We *Want* to Do?

A. *Take an honest review of what we* want *to do.* For the church it is most likely that we want to protect and support all those who are called to work in and for the church, treating everyone with compassion and respect for their dignity. In order to accomplish this in an era of HIV and AIDS may require that the organizational functions of the church are modified appropriately to reflect and respond to the reality of HIV within the church, and to mitigate the impact of AIDS on staff and church functioning, both now and in the future.

What can we do to respond to those factors that are likely to increase vulnerability to HIV infection and how can we mitigate the impacts of HIV and AIDS? How can we minimize the effect of HIV and AIDS on the church and its work?

Armed with better understanding of the implications of HIV and AIDS for both those working in the church and the functioning of the church, it is possible to work together to identify different ways to address risks, vulnerabilities, and impacts and to find ways of increasing the coping capacity at all levels.

Dialogue is an essential key in order to ensure the responses are appropriare, are relevant, and create a sense of ownership. Explore together the different options for responding to decrease the risk and vulnerability, including all areas of prevention, care, and support for staff. Find ways to work together on the potential impacts of HIV and AIDS, to identify what coping capacities are already in place, what capacities are needed, and what responses would best help them to be aware of risks and to minimize the impact.

B. *Do no harm.* There are situations and ways in which employees may be made more susceptible to the risk of HIV infection by virtue of working for the church. These will have been identified (see the section on "Where Are We Now?") and it may be necessary to alter the current systems and ways of working to reduce and avoid putting people in situations that increase their vulnerability. This may involve capacity building, fresh training, new skills, redeployment of staff, flexible hours, keeping families together in duty postings, fair wages, clear forms of regular support, and so forth. Always actively seek to address the structural gender imbalances that are driving HIV.

Int. Ms. 4: What Can We Do?

Start by reflecting on the mission, mandate, goals, and core functions of the church, especially in relation to employees and their overall vulnerability to HIV. It is essential to create an enabling environment for the support, care, and treatment of all employees in the era of HIV. The following are key areas on which the church can focus that are appropriate and can make a significant difference.

A. *Development of a church HIV and AIDS workplace policy.* One of the most important and helpful responses is the development of a "workplace policy" in line with national policy and legislation. Such a policy is a clear statement of commitment on the way the church or institution will respond to HIV and AIDS within the workplace and is based on accepted decisions made by the same church or institution. The development and implementation of such a policy requires consultation with and involvement of those who work in and for the church, especially with those already either living with the virus or personally affected. It should provide the framework for action, ensure consistency, and establish standards of behaviour for all church workers and the congregation, whether infected or not. It preempts inaction and enables difficult decisions on HIV and AIDS response. The church should not view the formulation of such a policy, particularly on HIV and AIDS, as an option, but as a responsibility to the people and a calling from God. Care must be taken to ensure that the policy is not developed to support or justify any current church programmes. Rather, it must provide guidelines for quality responses in the present and in the future.[13] All need to know of its existence and content and be able to readily access it. This leads to greater ownership, more commitment to the process of mitigating HIV in the workplace, and a greater likelihood the policy will be implemented.

First, review what policies and practices are currently in place in the church, particularly in the light of HIV. It may be necessary to revisit the policies or to develop specific church workplace policies on HIV and AIDS and on gender to ensure that there is a concerted effort to:

- State the church's position with regard to HIV and AIDS and those affected by the virus.
- State what the church is committed to do with regard to HIV and AIDS and all those affected.
- Acknowledge the risks of HIV.
- Improve understanding of the virus and the determinants to its spread.
- Address and reduce the susceptibility of church employees to HIV.
- Reduce the vulnerability of both the employees and the church, as an organization, to the impact of HIV and AIDS.
- Be gender-sensitive.
- Be in line with the national labour laws on HIV and AIDS, gender, and human rights.
- Formalize the responsibility of the church to its employees.

There are many useful examples of workplace policies that can be used as guidelines or templates that can be adapted. It is important, however, not to just copy another entity's policy document but to develop one that captures local input and is relevant to the particular context and denomination in which you are working. The guidelines below suggested by the International Labour Organisation are inclusive and comprehensive and may form a good basis for any church-based workplace-policy document.

International Labour Organisation (ILO):
Main Concept for a Workplace Policy Document

- Recognize HIV as a workplace issue
- Ensure nondiscrimination in the workplace
- Eradicate all forms of stigma and discrimination in all HIV interventions
- Ensure gender equality
- Aim to provide a healthy work environment and investigate and/or provide health and workplace insurances, which could include provision of ARVs
- Protect staff from vulnerability to infection
- Support staff who are living with HIV and ensure continuation of employment relationship
- Encourage social dialogue
- Promote HIV prevention, care, and support for all employees

- Ensure that the church does not increase the vulnerability of communities or undermine their coping options or strategies
- Respect confidentiality
- Involve people living with HIV

In addition, a policy document should include employment criteria, contain grievance procedures, and uphold nondiscrimination of all, irrespective of gender and HIV serostatus. HIV testing should not be a requirement or a prerequisite for hiring and/or continuation of employment. It is very helpful if such a document also includes a commitment to take disciplinary action against forms of stigma and discrimination and any sexual harassment.

Careful follow-up is necessary. There may be need to review and harmonize implications of HIV policy with other organizational policies.[14]

Such a policy should ultimately create an environment of mutual support and benefit ensuring a healthy, appreciated, and HIV-knowledgeable workforce able to cope with the challenges of HIV and AIDS and to accomplish the desired and planned activities of the church.

The following policy statement is an example that is comprehensive and inclusive of many sections, each of which, within the full policy document, is expanded with proposed activities and follow-up.

The HIV and AIDS Policy Statement—Catholic Church in Ethiopia

Commitment: "The HIV and AIDS epidemic will affect all the functions and services of the Ethiopian Catholic Church (ECC). Hence, our response to the epidemic is reflected to be part of all our services and functions."

1. The ECC as *Pastoral Minister*. This states that both the HIV-infected and affected retain all of their rights to participate in the life of the ECC, including the right to observe all the sacraments of the church and that the right to confidentiality will be upheld.

2. The ECC as *Employer*. This section affirms HIV-positive people to the right to equal employment opportunities and the church's obligation to ensure the protection of those rights. Included here are policies on: hiring; continued employment; education for ECC employees; confidentiality; psychosocial support; employee benefits; job modifications and accommodation; and medical coverage.

3. The ECC as *Educator*. This comprehensive section covers admission and continued enrollment in ECC schools—no testing requirements; education programmes about HIV and AIDS, TB, and all related issues including the gender dynamics and the impact of HIV; and practical recommendations to provide care and support in the school and community for school administrators, teachers, and parents on a regular basis. Instruction on the use of universal precautions in case of injuries will be provided. Stigma will be counteracted in every possible way. Education includes the laity and religious leaders and ensures confidentiality.

4. The ECC as a *Social Service Provider*. This section covers all the areas of social service provision.

5. The ECC for *Justice*. The ECC confirms its responsibility and obligation to promote justice on behalf of those living with HIV or in any way affected by AIDS.

6. *Policy implementation, networking, and coordination*. This section outlines the formulation of a national strategic framework and relevant guidelines for the implementation of policy.

B. *Appoint a focal person in the church.* While the overall responsibility for mainstreaming remains with the pastor or church leaders and with the programme/project heads, it is often very useful to delegate the practical coordination of the process to one person who may be called the focal person, or to a team of persons referred to as the focal point.[15] Leadership in the church or institution may already be over-burdened. Having someone who is specifically responsible to champion the issues, maintain confidentiality, and be the link-motivating person on HIV and AIDS issues in the church can improve the successful implementation of the process. This is dependent, however, on the degree of support the person receives, the extent of his or her mandate, and the continued involvement of everyone in addressing HIV in the church.

The focal person (FP) task should not be imposed—interest and commitment are prerequisites for being an effective FP. Focal persons should be recruited, trained, and assisted in addressing their own attitudes, stigmas, understandings, and misunderstandings as well as receiving the appropriate training for their position. They will have the responsibility of acting as a catalyst to mainstream HIV and AIDS activities within their sector as well as collaboration with other focal persons. They will also require mentoring and support and may at times need expert support. For the FP to be able to fulfill the tasks, the necessary human, financial, and material resources have to be made available.

Ideally, there should be a focal person at all levels. Even though the focal person will be leading the mainstreaming activities, it should not mean that all questions related to HIV and AIDS are delegated to this person. HIV and AIDS should remain everybody's business. Without effective teamwork toward the same goal and without the support of committed leadership and colleagues, the appointment of an HIV and AIDS Focal Person may even be counterproductive.

Advice for a New Focal Person[16]

- Find out what is expected of you in your new role as HIV and AIDS focal person.
- Start by having a meeting with your church leader and other key decision makers to explain the meaning and implications of mainstreaming HIV and AIDS. You will need their support in the future and they need to appreciate your new role and the responsibilities of a focal person.
- Carry out a desk study on HIV and AIDS mainstreaming to find out what has already happened in the church, what plans there are for the future, and who the key players are (include NGOs, donors, researchers, and others in your sector).
- Develop strategic alliances and support structures: talk to people with experience in HIV and AIDS responses both within and outside of the church (including NGOs, donors, researchers and HIV and AIDS, and focal persons in other churches and other sectors).
- Ensure that the work involved in mainstreaming HIV and AIDS is included in your job description.
- Seek support from all key stakeholders within and outside your department/ministry (this should include financial resources that are well targeted and/or earmarked).
- Build support amongst colleagues and peers.
- Seek practical support, for instance, office facilities and resources as well as any identified further relevant training.

C. *Programmes: Adapt, modify, redesign, and empower.* In order to mainstream HIV competence into the programmes, there is need to relook at what is currently been undertaken, in the light of the information collected in the various analysis above and in light of what is decided that should now be done. Programmes thus may need to be specific, adapted, modified, redesigned, or developed as a completely new initiative. Involvement in this development of both those who will work in the programme and those who benefit from it will ensure that the intention to decrease HIV risks and reduce vulnerabilities is addressed.

1. *Decrease HIV risks.* The most common activities that are developed to address the internal environment of any organization tend to focus on vulnerable groups, risky situations, and identified gaps in the current HIV activities.[17] The activities can do the following:

- Create a conducive environment that is open, nonstigmatizing, and free of HIV fears, where rights are promoted, staff feel supported and experience care, and their dignity is respected and upheld.
- Aim to reduce preventable risks through regular, well-informed, and open discussions; providing information, awareness, and training to address HIV and AIDS; and addressing gender-specific concerns in order to promote behaviour change amongst staff, partners, and beneficiaries. This should be done in a way that is gender-sensitive to the particular needs and different risks of men and women and should promote gender equality and equity at all levels.
- Ensure that the church is not contributing to risks.
- Ensure staff has access to necessary resources and services/referral systems for prevention, testing, counselling, treatment, care, and support. Create linkages with health services and others HIV-focused stakeholders who are providing necessary services and resources not currently available in the church.
- Ensure the meaningful involvement of people living with HIV to raise awareness and reduce stigma.
- Provide appropriate resource materials, HIV- and AIDS-focused literature, and access to up-to-date information; promote protective measures that are appropriate; peer education; make available and distribute appropriate resource material; promote the "SAVE" acronym in place of the stigmatizing "ABC" acronym.[18]
- Encourage confidential testing and provide access to or referral to family counselling, care, and treatment services.
- Establish support groups for HIV-positive employees and families.

2. *Minimize HIV impact on the functioning of the church.* In order to minimize the way HIV and AIDS affects the functioning of the church, there is need to modify the way the church functions in relation to its employees, so as to minimize the impact of AIDS on them as well as on the work of the church.

Engage in dialogue and work together with the employees in the church on the potential impacts of HIV and of AIDS on themselves and their families, to identify what coping capacities are already in place, what capacities are needed, and what responses would best help them to minimize the impact. Include all areas of prevention, care, and support for staff. Do not overlook the morale of people who work within the church. Loss of colleagues or the additional workload expected through multitasking may affect the general morale; this needs to be recognized and acknowledged, and the necessary support systems must be put in place, including specific support groups. Consider also establishing special funds or collections of material goods to help the most affected and those caring for additional children as a consequence of AIDS deaths or illness within families.

Investigate the possibilities of having health insurance plans provide for anti-retroviral therapy or encourage those working in the church to consider taking out their own insurance plans. Consider also the provision of disability and funeral benefits.

Identify the strengths already within the church workers to cope. Where there are identified gaps, seek to build their capacity to cope with and to mitigate the impact of HIV and AIDS.

Plan with workers on the process and the targets needed to accomplish these tasks, as this allows for self-measurement of progress and of change. Learn from the process, adapt where necessary, capture good practices, and share experiences encountered in the process.

3. *Mitigate against financial implications.* Be aware of the financial implications for the church and adapt as appropriate, particularly in relation to the provision of additional services and support systems, employment of relief workers, additional training and supervision, and the financial implications related to the full implementation of the workplace policy.

HIV and AIDS require a specific budget line. This needs to be built into the budget lines for the operation of the church at the onset of every financial cycle. Additional resources may need to be raised, if not locally then from donors.

4. *Build capacity and form strategic partnerships.* Build the capacity of those who work in the church through training programmes, exposure visits, support groups, and any other strategy that is identified as helpful and necessary, especially to implement the agreed-upon activities.

Encourage networks within and between churches that are already involved in mainstreaming HIV and form strategic partners with the many service providers with expertise and focused interventions on HIV and AIDS. It is not always possible to do everything, nor is it advisable. Take advantage of the services provided by others and make them aware of the services that you offer.

Look toward forming partnerships with people living with HIV and the various networks in which they are involved. Their experiences can help inform the relevancy of the processes and ensure that stigma is excluded. The World Council of Churches, together with INERELA+ and UNAIDS, have developed various resource materials and toolkits to assist in such a partnership.

Int. Ms. 5: Implement and Document

Implementation of the various solutions and strategies will require modifying the way things have usually been done, in order to take into account the reality of HIV and AIDS. Such changes require commitment and buy-in from all concerned, for the sake of all concerned.

Document the process, the networking opportunities and results, and the outcome of all actions. It is a way of confirming that the process is on track, provides a template for replication, and is a record for institutional memory.

Int. Ms. 6: Monitor and Evaluate Progress, Learn, and Share

At the time of planning, decide what you want the outcome to be as a result of the planned activities and modified ways of doing things. This will be the benchmark against which you can measure progress.

Measure and evaluate the progress of implementation, especially of the workplace policy and the altered running of the church functions, learn from the outcomes, and adapt as appropriate. Learn from the experiences and share with others; transferring knowledge and experiences leads to scale-up.

Summary: Internal Mainstreaming

Internal mainstreaming is about recognizing and acknowledging the reality of HIV—susceptibility, risks, and vulnerability—in the lives of those who serve in the church, and proactively working to reduce these risks. It is also measuring the current impact and predicting the potential impact and introducing or changing policies and practices in order to limit risks and to mitigate the impacts.

Ultimately, such internal mainstreaming should result in transformed, motivated, and supported employees and a church that is strengthened in its response to HIV and AIDS in its internal domain.

Core Features
Internal Mainstreaming HIV and AIDS Competence

1. **What is our vision?**

2. **Where are we now?**

   ### 2.1 Organizational Analysis
   - How are those who work in and for the church affected by HIV and AIDS?
     - Risks—what is putting people at risk?
     - Vulnerabilities—what is increasing their vulnerabilities?
   - Any policies/strategies/resources available to respond?

   ### 2.2 Impact Assessment
   - The impact of HIV and AIDS on:
     - Those who work in and for the church
     - The work of the church

3. **What do we *want* to do?**
   - Protect and support staff of the church
   - Modify the organizational functions of the church to:
     - Reflect the reality of HIV and AIDS within the church
     - Limit and mitigate the impact of AIDS on staff and church functioning
   - Ensure that we do no harm: do not increase people's risks and vulnerability to HIV by virtue of their working in and for the church

4. **What *can* we do?**
   - Workplace policy
   - Appoint focal person
   - Programmes: specific and adapted
   - Build capacity and form partnerships

5. **Implement and document**

6. **Monitor and evaluate progress, learn and share**

5.5 External Mainstreaming:
The External Domain of the Church

The external domain of the church refers to the areas or domain in which the church carries out its activities both within the church itself and in the communities. External mainstreaming means ensuring that an HIV response is made part of the core function of the church, its activities, projects, and programmes. It ensures the activities undertaken with congregations and communities are suitably adapted to take into account the reality that everyone may be susceptible to HIV infection and vulnerable to the impact of both HIV and AIDS, and it should include care for those most affected. These activities must also reflect a gender perspective, for without addressing this dimension, we do not adequately address one of the biggest drivers of the epidemic. As in the situation of internal mainstreaming, external mainstreaming should reflect the church's mission, mandate, objectives, and core functions. These activities should complement the local and national strategic plans on HIV and AIDS.

Keep people at the centre in all that is done. Effective mainstreaming of HIV and AIDS requires leadership, networking, and forming partnerships.

If the church is to be really relevant and to make a significant difference in the arena of HIV, then it is imperative to recognize the key drivers of the virus, especially contextually. It means identifying risks and vulnerabilities and the knowledge and skills of our target groups as to these risks and where to find help and support. It also involves an honest look at our own skills, knowledge, and availability of the appropriate partners and resources (structural, financial, human, material, and spiritual) to respond appropriately, compassionately, and ultimately to make a positive difference in the quality of lives by reducing the spread of HIV, mitigating the impact of AIDS and ultimately restoring hope and dignity.

The people who work in this domain, the "staff," do need to have developed inner HIV competence in terms of understanding, attitudes, knowledge, and inner conviction on the necessity and rationale for mainstreaming HIV, so that there is common understanding of the process. They may require appropriate training, continuous accurate information, and capacity building in order to be better equipped to mainstream HIV and AIDS in the activities (see section 4, above). It also ensures they are proactively seeking opportunities for engagement with communities and adaptation of their usual work to respond to the real needs and concerns of the communities.

The principles of external mainstreaming include:

- Identifying and responding to factors within the context that are likely to increase risk and vulnerability to HIV infection for the individuals and communities with whom the church works.
- Ensuring that the work of the church is not increasing the vulnerability to HIV infection or impacts of AIDS of those for whom it is working or undermining their options for coping with the affects of the pandemic.
- Recognizing the likely impacts of HIV and AIDS on those with whom the church works and the community with which it works.
- Identifying the comparative advantage of the church and the contributions it can make to respond to HIV and AIDS, including preempting, reversing, or mitigating impacts and improving the lives of those most affected.

The following is a suggested process that can be followed to ensure HIV is adequately and appropriately mainstreamed into the external domain of the church.

Ext. Ms. 1: Vision

Identify, with the community members, what they would like their community to look like without risks, now, in a couple of years, and for the long-term future. Can they envisage the possibility of an AIDS-free generation, where stigma is contained, no infants are born HIV-positive, all people are sufficiently aware and empowered that there be no new HIV infections, and nobody dies of AIDS-related illnesses because of inability to access the needed services, care, support, and treatment? Moreover, might it be possible to ensure there is also zero tolerance to all forms of gender violence, particularly sexual gender-based violence? What might be the barriers to that vision or dream becoming a reality and what would be needed to realize that vision for the community? *If a community has a clear vision, wants it badly enough, and is committed to realize the vision, it can happen.* If it is their vision, they own the responses and can build on the strengths already present and active in the community. It moves away from the notion of just being trapped in a situation to realizing that there may well be possibilities, within the capabilities of the community, to address the risks, reduce vulnerabilities, and cushion the impact of AIDS. It also opens the possibilities for communities to both realize and advocate for their own basic human rights, especially in relation to HIV and its impact.

Together develop a vision for this process. For example:

HIV and AIDS competence is competently mainstreamed into all the activities of the church and its ministries, taking into account the reality that everyone is susceptible to HIV infection, the risks are much greater for some than others, and all may be vulnerable to the impact of both HIV and AIDS. Activities may need to be adapted to significantly decrease the risks of HIV infection, minimize vulnerabilities, and mitigate the impact, thus improving the lives of all, especially people already living with HIV.

Ext. Ms. 2: Where Are We Now?

In order to achieve our vision, we need to assess where we are now and gain a deeper understanding of the way HIV and AIDS are affecting the people with whom we work and the community in which they live. Thus it is necessary to collect some baseline community data: a context analysis and an impact assessment. Some of the information may already be available from national statistics and from other partners working in the same communities.

Ext. Ms. 2.1: Context Analysis

Identify the presence of HIV, the key drivers of the epidemic, and the ways HIV and AIDS have affected and continue to affect the people we work with, and the responses.

Key information to be collected may include the following:[19]

A. *General HIV and AIDS situation.* Ascertain HIV prevalence in these communities. This information may be available from the national statistics or, if more localized, can be guided by seroprevalence rates and frequency of HIV-related illnesses in the community as identified in local health facilities; availability and size of support groups; frequency of funerals; and so forth.

B. *Risks and vulnerabilities.*

- Explore the basic understanding of HIV and AIDS and the prevailing attitudes, beliefs, fears, and prejudices about HIV and the extent of stigma and discrimination. Does the community recognize HIV as a problem and discuss it openly?
- What factors are contributing to the spread of HIV and increasing vulnerability to HIV infection amongst specific groups, including women, youth, and communities?
- What is the level of knowledge among the community members regarding the risks, the determinants of the risks, and where to find information and/ or help? Do community members understand the linkage between the risk and HIV infection, such as how rape increases the chance of HIV infection?

- Note the extent of the populations' movement.
- Explore and seek to understand some of the priority concerns, which may represent risks to HIV infection, that are being faced by members of the community, according to context, age, gender, culture, and current situation. Note how these risks are affecting them and having an impact on their lives (for instance, peer pressure and coercion; communication difficulties and lack of skills in marital conflict management; lack of access to correct information or services; abuse, including sexual abuse; gender-based violence; drugs; and cultural factors that facilitate the transmission of HIV).
- Which social groups in the community are more vulnerable and more affected by HIV and AIDS? Do we have families that are "invisible" to us because they are so badly affected and no longer participate in activities? These are priority groups who will require special attention.
- Seek to understand the vulnerability of members of the community to the risks and how to cope. The presence of risks in the community does not automatically make people vulnerable but certain situations may definitely increase their vulnerability to HIV infection such as: unsupervised youth; orphans without responsible caregivers; lack of support structures— a "shoulder to cry on";[20] risky environment such as unlit pathways from transport routes and beer halls en route to schools; poverty, which affects choices; alcohol excess in home environment; and so forth.

C. *Current responses and coping mechanisms.* HIV and AIDS are already in the communities and are already being responded to in one way or another. It is important to discover how they are being dealt with and what can be built upon. Communities have innate strengths and coping mechanisms, though frequently these are not exercised nor are communities given opportunity to tap into them. Explore together these skills and strengths and see how they are being used to:

- Identify risks;
- Reduce risks and address the threat of HIV;
- Prevent HIV (for instance, access to preventative strategies and services; life-skills and assertiveness training; provision of support structures such as a "shoulder to cry on"; legal protection; safe spaces);
- Mitigate against impact and receive support if impacted;
- Establish whether the community engages with people living with HIV in any sustained way;
- Determine gaps in the current response and opportunities for improving or scaling up.

D. *Stakeholder analysis and availability of social services.* Assess who is doing what, where, how, when, and with whom in response to HIV and AIDS, especially within the community served by the church. Map services, both within the church and in the surrounding community, that are available and can be called upon, referred to, or used as sources of information and assistance. Examples: health-care points, local clinics, and opportunistic infection services; home-based care; local NGOs working in the field of HIV; testing centres; counselling services; legal aid services; and so forth.

- Who is doing what and where and how effectively?
- Is the community aware of these services and where and how to access them?
- Are the services offered in a nondiscriminatory and stigma-free environment?
- Also, within any congregation, there are likely to be professional people such as doctors, nurses, and counselors who may be willing to be called upon to give advice or do programme direction. Do we know who they are, whether or not they would be willing to be involved, and whether they are given the opportunity to be involved in our programmes and outreaches?

E. *Availability of policies/instruments/resources (financial, human, structural, technical, spiritual).* Investigate what policies and other helpful documents or instruments have already been developed, are available, or are currently in use. These may form the basis of future activities and can be further developed, modified, or adapted as may be required under the process of mainstreaming.

Ext. Ms. 2.2: Impact Assessment

A. *Impact of HIV and AIDS on those with whom we work (beneficiaries and the community)*

- Note the consequences or impacts of HIV and AIDS on the community's morbidity, mortality, health-care demands, orphanhood, AIDS-induced poverty, stigma, and discrimination.
- Estimate the impacts of HIV and AIDS, both social and economic, in the medium to long term. Is HIV causing changes in the socioeconomic context and livelihoods by deepening poverty, and is this reflected in increasing illness, loss, and death; increasing numbers of children who are orphaned; noticeable school dropouts; an increased burden of care on women and girls; and a reduction in food security? Are extended families no longer reliable social networks, especially for children orphaned by AIDS? How are the HIV-related illnesses, AIDS deaths, and stigma affecting the communities?
- Does the community have the knowledge and skills to deal with the impact and do they know where to find help? How effective is this response?

B. *Assess the impact of HIV and AIDS on those who work in and for the church, and thus on the work of the church, within the communities served.* Examples of such impacts include the following:

- The load of pastoral care increases exponentially.
- Staff capacity may be limited due to repeated illnesses, leading to poorer quality in work and decreased morale and motivation.
- There are more frequent funerals than baptisms in areas of high prevalence.
- There are increasing numbers of orphans needing support.
- There is an increased financial burden on the church with ever-increasing demands for help and support.
- The availability of volunteers becomes unreliable because of their own domestic demands due to the impact of HIV at home.
- The church expects a decreased income in collections and donations as affected families, with the increasing financial demands because of HIV, have less disposable income.
- On the positive side, the church may receive increased donor funding to enable it to respond to a greater scale and more effectively to the impact of AIDS.

Ext Ms. 3: What Do We *Want* to Do?

A. *Involve the community.* In every situation, there is the danger of viewing it from an "us" and "them" perspective, meaning that there is the danger of seeing "ourselves" as the experts and "the other" as people in need of our solutions, based upon our external perceptions of their experience rather than engaging to learn with them. We may tend to overlook their strengths and coping capacities and instead focus on perceived needs. In order to truly learn and to bridge the us-them divide by opening the space between us for cross-learning and sharing, we need first to listen with an open mind, appreciate current efforts, and hear from the communities what they feel could make a more positive difference in their lives. They can best share both how HIV and AIDS are affecting them, as it is their lived reality, and what they see as the key drivers of the epidemic within the context in which they are experiencing its implications.

If the community is involved in identifying what the current situation is and what they would hope it might be with appropriate interventions, and if they are involved in identifying and designing innovative solutions, there is far more local ownership of the process, less reliance on outside assistance, and a greater likelihood of more local monitoring of the process as it unfolds.

In addition, such community initiatives can give the people a sense of purpose and ownership and, above all, a sense of hope that something *can* be done.[21]

> Communities, with the right knowledge, skills, and approach,
> have the capacity to solve their own problems. After all, these are
> their practices and traditions. Who are we, as outsiders with our
> limited understandings and appreciation, to try to get involved
> beyond the role of catalysts? Instead, we must use these opportu-
> nities to learn so that our future materials are based on evidence
> and less on assumptions. —*Louis Chingander*[22]

B. *Do no harm.* While acknowledging the good we may do, which is often more obvious, we also need to consider the potential negative implications of what we do. How could the activities currently being undertaken or planned by the church/institution actually contribute to the spread of HIV and increase vulnerability to infection? Are our activities actually undermining individual or community coping capacities? Are vulnerable people included, regardless of their HIV status? For example:

- All-night prayer vigils and funeral wakes, or camps for youth, may offer opportunities for clandestine sexual activities that are unprotected and increase risk of HIV transmission.
- Trainings offered by the church/institution may separate families for the duration of the training, or may have costs involved that put a strain on the resources of the affected households.
- Trainings offered may be held at a considerable distance from the homes of the participants, thus putting them at risk when walking/travelling. Similarly, if the trainings finish late, the participants will be returning home in the dark.
- School fees in our education institutions may be beyond the reach of some and pupils who cannot afford the fees may be vulnerable to exploitation from those with the needed resources, resulting in exchanging sex for fees.
- In our church schools, pupils may not be receiving sufficient or appropriate training in sex and reproductive health, as well as life skills, to deal with the responsibility of their sexuality and that of the other. Pupils may thus not be equipped to be able to assert themselves and to say no to coercion. Younger pupils may be exploited by sexually active older pupils or staff; specific measures need to be in place for staff as well.
- Clinic and hospital user fees may be out of the reach of some affected households, who may either not access much-needed care or increase their vulnerability by draining their remaining resources.
- Staff may be separated from their spouses for long periods of time.

- HIV-positive medical staff may conceal their status if they fear stigmatization, loss of employment, or other unfair labour practices. They may be tempted to steal drugs.
- In development work, we may site schools, boreholes, and toilets without considering whether accessing them will increase the risk of the user(s), especially women and children, to personal dangers and thus to HIV infection.
- The programmes may foster gender inequalities in the allocation of posts or authority structures and thus create opportunities for abuse or exploitation of the beneficiaries.
- People living with HIV may be excluded from job opportunities and in-service benefits.
- In high-prevalence areas, some people may be excluded from programmes because of perceived risks to the staff.

Ext. Ms. 4: What *Can* We Do?

Start with the opportunities and strengths already demonstrated and seek to acknowledge and enhance these before recognizing the gaps and barriers and threats. This is important so that one is not overwhelmed by a sense of helplessness in being able to do anything in the way of protection or mitigation, in light of the contextual realities in which some people find themselves.

A. *Identify the comparative advantage of the church.* The church has a huge comparative advantage over other sectors, as has already been described in section 3.1, when it comes to local credibility, presence, practices, mandate, and potential. Where human resources are involved, the church is unparalleled in terms of the variety and sheer numbers within its ranks who could be called upon as volunteers, who could give advice as professionals, or who are already working within the church. The church has many partners and links from grassroots to the international communities. It has people living with HIV and people very affected by HIV within its domain who bring the lived reality to the discussions and who may contribute significantly to the development of an appropriate HIV and AIDS response.

There are many technical tools and resources available to guide processes as well as several NGOs working in the same field with experiences to share. Financial resources can be found.

Review what policies, strategies, and actions are already in place that can be modified or adapted to meet the prevailing needs and prevent or mitigate negative impacts.

Most of all, unlike secular organizations with sectoral responses to HIV and AIDS, the church seeks to bring about transformation in people's lives, restoring relationships between the individual and God, and between individuals and their fellow humans. This also involves a restoration in relationship with oneself—reclaiming a belief in one's own value and innate potential. A transformed person seeks a higher good and the common good of mankind and seeks to change that which is detrimental to achieving this.

B. *Adapt programmes/design or redesign programmes/target the most vulnerable/empower communities.* The context analysis should precede the planning of mainstreaming activities. Such an analysis should address both the causes of HIV (the "upstream" causes of HIV) and the implications of HIV and AIDS (the "downstream" effects) on beneficiaries, services, and policies. These analyses assist in identifying the causes and barriers to achieving our identified vision for the church and community. The combined knowledge—context analysis and implications assessment—forms the basis for re/designing and adapting programmes in order to integrate relevant activities that address and reduce risk, minimize vulnerability, and mitigate against impacts related to HIV and AIDS. It is important that activities target especially the most vulnerable, such as households with sick members, widows and the elderly, child-headed households, food-insecure households, and so forth. By actively and proactively seeking to empower individuals and communities, the responses become more relevant and self-sustaining. Plan together to:

- Prioritize risks based on risk assessment and identified needs.
- Redesign programmes to integrate activities to address knowledge barriers, risks, vulnerabilities, and impact mitigation wherever necessary. Ensure our work helps (and does not hinder) them to be less susceptible to the identified risks and less vulnerability to the impact of AIDS.

C. *Decrease risks and minimize vulnerability factors.* Some of the activities that can be done include the following:

- Adapt programmes to respond appropriately to the reality of HIV risks and vulnerabilities as identified in the baseline survey.
- HIV and AIDS programmes: This may include the introduction of specific programmes on HIV and AIDS if they do not already exist, or it may involve adapting the programmes to make them more relevant to reducing the susceptibility of individuals and communities to HIV infection.
- Behaviour-change programmes, peer education, and trainings to increase HIV awareness and knowledge of HIV and all the key factors associated with its transmission, prevention, key drivers, linkage with development issues, treatment and care, and support.
- Encourage "Know your status"—confidential counselling and testing.
- Promote access to services and support programmes.
- Breakdown stigma, discrimination, and associated inequities.

D. *Recognize, preempt, reverse, and mitigate impact.*

- Target the most vulnerable, such as the elderly, sick, widows, child-headed households, households with sick members, orphans and vulnerable children, and food-insecure households, and ensure they are part of all programmes. Ensure the programmes meet their needs rather than ours.
- Empowerment programmes are the key to sustainability and moving people away from dependency.
- Ensure there are policies to overcome gender inequalities and inequities.
- Encourage self-reliance programmes for people living with HIV.
- Poverty-reduction programmes can make a critical difference where the impact of AIDS is most noticeable.

Thus, while maintaining the core functions of our programmes, reexamine the current approach and modify where necessary to meet specific needs of people living with HIV and affected homes, to improve their lives and those of the communities and to ensure that neither the communities we serve, nor the staff, are at risk of HIV infection.

E. *Build capacity and form strategic partnerships.* Identify skills needed by the leadership and the community and acquire the necessary training, resources, toolkits, and collaboration in order to be equipped appropriately to deal with the prioritized risks. In addition, consider developing a curriculum that will include these prioritized challenges to ensure they are addressed in the overall programme. Give these challenges the importance and the time allocation appropriate to the significance of the issues.

Ongoing accurate information should be provided. By empowering communities, sustainability is more likely in the long run.

For the most effective implementation, the church should seek out partners and establish strategic relationships with key stakeholders whose interventions focus on HIV and AIDS. This enlarges the potential for additional funding sources and technical assistance and enables the establishment of a sound referral system, especially with those who offer services that deal with abuse cases, counselling services, testing, treatment, support groups, and the like. We cannot do everything ourselves, but so much more can be achieved collaboratively. Be sure to inform such partners of the activities the church is doing for mutual collaboration and strength and sharing of good practices.

Example: "A church working with young people wants to prevent the spread of HIV among young people in its town. Through one of its programmes, the church works directly with young people in school, so that they have the help and education that they need to reduce their risk of HIV infection. Through one of its partnerships, the church works with key people in the Ministry of Education, so that they might support sexual health education in schools. The church's partnership is helping to improve the overall environment in which other churches and NGOs work and in which young people protect themselves from HIV."

F. *What church issues affect partnerships?*[23] The views that others have of a church can also make it difficult to build partnerships. Partners may not know about the church or understand a church's positive role. For example:

- A businessperson may think that a church lacks credibility because not-for-profit organizations do not operate with the "reality" of market forces.
- A donor may receive so many requests from different churches and NGOs, making it hard to distinguish one from the other.
- A organization for people living with HIV may view your church negatively due to issues such as prevention or stigmatization.

Church issues to consider when building partnerships include the following:

- Negative images of churches. Partners may think that churches cannot be trusted to get results, or that they will create problems by refusing to face difficult issues.
- Perceptions about a church's resources. Partners may underestimate, or overestimate, what a church can do.
- A church's reputation. Partners may seek out only the most prominent churches, or avoid ones that are thought of as too "vocal" or "fringe."
- Balance with other areas of a church's work. Partnerships can consume much time and take away energy needed for programme activities.
- Competition among churches. Partnerships can create an atmosphere of tension or mistrust among other churches and NGOs.
- The dynamics of gender, class, age, sexual orientation, and economic context in their projects and programmes.

Example of an Effective Partnership: Church Health Association of Zambia (CHAZ)

Established in 1970, CHAZ is an umbrella organization of church (Catholic and Protestant) health institutions and community-based organizations. It is the second-largest health-care provider in Zambia, accounting for approximately 50 percent of rural area coverage.

CHAZ-member health facilities operate on a not-for-profit basis and within the policy framework of the Ministry of Health whose vision is to: "provide equity of access to cost-effective, quality health care as close to the family as possible." Through a memorandum of understanding (MOU) between the government and

CHAZ, these health facilities have full government support for human resources, grants for running costs, and essential drugs. This MOU has been effectively operating since the 1980s and makes CHAZ a worthy recipient of donor money aimed at country ownership and sustainability of large-scale health programs, including HIV-related care and treatment.

The organization has had many strategic alliances over the years with different cooperating partners taking health services and general community development to all provinces of Zambia. Over the last 24 years, CHAZ has worked with and successfully subgranted funds from a number of development and global partners, including the government of the Republic of Zambia (GRZ), the World Health Organization Global Program for AIDS (WHO/GPA), NORAD, DanChurchAid (DCA), the European Union (EU), Family Health International (FHI), CORDAID, UNICEF, USAID, CIDA (Canada) the Royal Netherlands Embassy, Irish Aid, AIDS Relief (PEPFAR), and the Centre for Disease Control (CDC).

CHAZ boasts a strong supply-chain management system which is considered to be an integral component of the national supply-chain system. CHAZ has a presence in every province and its role as lead Civil Society Organization (CSO) in health-service delivery is evidence of the institution's vast experience and good understanding of CSOs in Zambia.

Due to CHAZ's extensive infrastructure and local experience managing the implementation of health programs which aim to make significant inroads into the disease burden in Zambia, the Zambia Country Coordinating Mechanism (CCM) chose CHAZ in 2002 to be one of the four principal recipients to disburse funds in Zambia. CCM-Zambia mandated CHAZ to disburse Global Fund money to faith-based organizations (Christian, Muslim, Baha'i, and Hindu) and oversee the implementation of HIV/AIDS, tuberculosis, and malaria activities through a grant from the Global Fund to fight those diseases. Since May 2003, CHAZ has successfully managed over $140 million dollars (US).

CHAZ has experienced much growth and has performed well in recent years. This development and exemplary performance is due in part to the competency and commitment of the secretariat staff coupled with the confidence CHAZ has cultivated among the donor community. This in turn is supported by CHAZ's transparent nature in accounting for donor funds and robust internal systems which ensure that funds given to CHAZ are used for the intended purposes: to benefit poor people, particularly in rural and hard-to-reach areas where church hospitals are located. This success story is also attributed to the support CHAZ receives from the government of the Republic of Zambia, the CHAZ board, managing churches and their leaders, church health facilities, and other implementing partner FBOs.

Ext. Ms. 5: Implement and Document

Once the action plan has been decided upon, together with the community, implement the agreed programme. It is also useful to:

- Establish clear responsibilities: Who does what, by when, and how?
- Determine accountability: To whom, how often, and how?
- Determine coordination mechanisms.
- Assess resources: What resources are available or required, including human and financial resources?
- Document: With implementation much is learned along the way. It is important that all activities and responses and subsequent changes noted are well documented. It is a way of ensuring that mainstreaming HIV is actually being carried out across our programmes and describes how the programme may be replicated and what pitfalls to avoid. Documentation also ensures institutional memory.

Ext. Ms. 6: Learn and Share: Transfer Knowledge and Experience

Share the learned experiences and the best practices with the people involved in the programmes and with other stakeholders, including donors. It can be very motivating and demonstrates accountability.

Ext. Ms. 7: Monitor and Evaluate Progress

Evaluate progress in relation to the agreed targets and plans and undertake frequent self-assessments of progress. Reevaluate the risks and impacts and see if there is need to change anything. It is only when we stand back from our activities and take a critical look at what we are doing, how we are doing it, with whom, why we are doing it, and with what are we doing it that we can honestly assess if we are actually making any difference.

Just as HIV is a dynamic epidemic, so also should our responses be dynamic. It can never be "business as usual" if we are to respond appropriately and effectively. As such, mainstreaming can never be viewed as a one-off event, but it remains an ongoing process.

Self-Assessment Checklist: Mainstreaming HIV[24]

Successful mainstreaming of HIV in a project means that it:

- Reaches its core objectives.
- Removes barriers and enables people living with HIV and affected people to participate in and derive benefits from the project activities.

- Minimizes the potential risks of HIV transmission and the impacts of HIV on beneficiary groups, staff, and volunteers.
- Enables or facilitates linkages to appropriate HIV services.
- Builds the capacity for analysis and intervention at all levels.
- Generates and uses evidence to improve our own work and influence the policy and practice environment in which we work.

Summary: External Mainstreaming

Core Features
External Mainstreaming HIV and AIDS Competence

1. **What is our vision?**
2. **Where are we now?**
   2.1 **Context analysis**
      - General HIV and AIDS situation in context
        - Risks
        - Vulnerabilities
        - Current responses, coping mechanisms, and involvement of people living with HIV
        - Stakeholder analysis and availability of social services
        - Availability of policies/instruments/resources (financial, human, structural, technical, spiritual, etc.)
   2.2 **Impact assessment:**
      - Impact of HIV and AIDS on those we work with (beneficiaries and the community)
        - Morbidity/mortality
        - Socioeconomic impact
        - Orphans and vulnerable children
        - Other impacts noted
      - Impact of HIV and AIDS on those who work in/for the church and thus on the work of the church, in the communities served
3. **What do we *want* to do?**
      - *Involve the communities so that the overall vision is jointly realized*
      - *Do no harm:* Ensure that the activities of the church do not increase the vulnerability to HIV infection of the people and communities with whom we work, or undermine their options for coping with the affects of the pandemic
4. **What *can* we do?**
      - Identify comparative advantage of the church
      - Adapt programmes/redesign/target most vulnerable/empower
        - Decrease risks
        - Minimize vulnerability
        - Mitigate impact
        - Capacity build and form strategic partnerships
5. **Implement and document**
6. **Learn. Share. Transfer knowledge and experience**
7. **Monitor and evaluate progress**

Summary Chart: Process of Mainstreaming HIV and AIDS Competence[25]

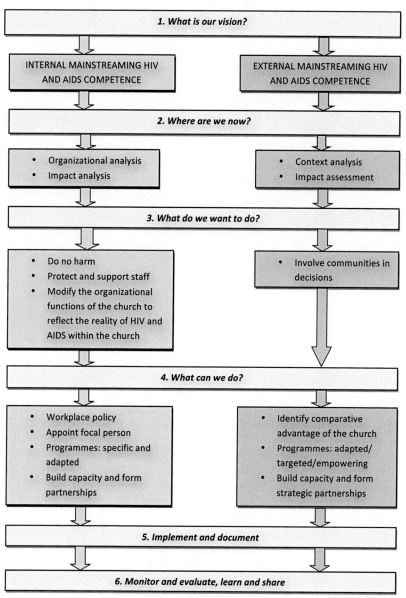

Parry Chart 5.1

Section 6
Mainstreaming HIV into Theological Institutions

HIV and AIDS trainings and programmes have tended to focus on the religious leaders who are already deployed in ministry. Since 2000, MAP International, the World Council of Churches, and others have sought to establish an effective way of reaching those still in training to view all their theological trainings through the eyes of HIV and AIDS. Too many pastors, ministers, and priests had expressed their sense of inadequacies in facing the multiple challenges raised by HIV and AIDS in the context in which they found themselves working. It was thus decided to develop tools to mainstream HIV and AIDS into the curricula of theological institutions and practically into all programmes, wherever such training was taking place. This process introduced discussions on the wider issues and key determinants of the spread of HIV. It involved writing, rewriting, and designing courses that tackled such subjects as: human sexuality and HIV; breaking the silence and finding language to address taboo subjects on sexuality; reading the Bible, especially the book of Job and the Gospels through the eyes of HIV; African theology and HIV; teaching the Bible, theology, and ethics in the context of HIV; counselling and accompaniment; gender justice and sexual and gender-based violence; skills to address the impact of AIDS in terms of orphans and elderly caregivers; deepening poverty; home-based care; project design and management; and many other emerging issues as the epidemic and responses to it have progressed. Those who would be on the frontline or who interface with communities grappling with the realities of HIV in their everyday life should be adequately informed and well prepared to respond with compassion and knowledge, showing leadership and accompaniment, and to restore dignity and hope to all who are affected by HIV and its devastating impact. This process has been ongoing; many resources have been developed to accompany theological institutions in this process and, to date, over 800 theological institutions across Africa have taken up the challenge.[1]

Mainstreaming HIV Competence into the Ministry of the Church

The previous sections have sought to describe what mainstreaming HIV and AIDS competence is all about: the essential principles, the questions to be answered, and the processes. The following sections explore the practice—the "how" of mainstreaming HIV competence into each section and ministry of the church. Each section presents a summary of key factors needed by those in specific leadership positions, responding to mainstreaming HIV and AIDS, in specific areas of the church's ministry.

The same process can be extended to the many institutions and sectors run by the church such as the education sector, health sector, the developmental arm, and many other activities in which the church is critically involved. Resources on mainstreaming into these and other similar specific sectors do exist, within the secular world, and thus will not be included here in any depth. However, the principles and processes remain the same. This section looks specifically at "the church."

It is not a comprehensive list and it is nonexhaustive. Interaction with the different sectors or groups below will reveal the specifics needed for that group. It must be contextual and address the challenges that *they* are facing in *their* context. The challenges faced may change between the sectors but there will nevertheless be cross-cutting issues that need to be explored. Find the appropriate techniques to deal with these. Because the ages and the genders of the groups will differ, there is need for age- and gender-sensitive and appropriate skills, always showing respect.

People who serve within the various departments of the church need both inner and outer competence in their respective areas of work and service. Many of them may be volunteers; nevertheless, it is incumbent on the responsible authorities in the church to have considered knowledge of all staff, whether employed or volunteers, and to establish an understanding of their attitudes, motivation, and appropriate skills. In the era of HIV, many contentious issues may arise, and the credibility of the whole church can be seriously compromised by the activities or responses of even one ill-informed or wrongly appointed worker. There is need to protect beneficiaries, the staff, and the church by ensuring that there is appropriate groundwork covered and necessary documentation in place as well as sufficient understanding and/or training of the potential worker.

For example: it is not merely enough to have someone willing to teach Bible stories to children; he or she must also be sufficiently prepared to understand and deal appropriately with situations that may arise as a consequence of HIV. What if those children are HIV-positive and there is a problem of acceptance by the other children? What if the child is a victim of sexual abuse? What if the child's experiences at home do not match the messages of love that we preach? Where was God for them when they lost someone they depended on and loved? How do they handle hearing from an ill-informed teacher that their loved relative died because "AIDS is a punishment from God"?

Infection with HIV does not "just happen." It is the end result of a long, complex process, a process of gender scripting and understanding, of attitudes, value systems, assertive skills, rights and responsibilities, choices, vulnerabilities, injustices, inequalities, violence, and many other life events. The church has the opportunity to engage at so many levels in this process: affirming the value of each and every one; empowering people; raising awareness; and giving people skills to identify their problems, understand consequences, make informed choices and take considered decisions, and advocate for equitable access to quality services and life-saving medications. The church also can work toward reducing vulnerabilities of communities and mitigating against the impact of AIDS.

Mainstreaming HIV into the life and ministry of the church gives the church the unique opportunity to accompany congregants from the youngest age through all the significant stages of development and events in life, and to intervene with appropriate knowledge, advice, and skills training at critical times in the life of the congregant. If this process is made uniform in all the churches, movement between churches or relocation will not matter, as the principle of responding to HIV seriously, appropriately, effectively, comprehensively, and compassionately will remain the same.

7.1 Church Leadership's Role in Mainstreaming HIV Issues
Leadership Must "Go Deeper"

> Let the wise learn and add to their learning, and let the discerning
> get guidance. —*Proverbs 1:5*

Leaders, true leaders, inspire others to believe in themselves and their ability to bring about change. When it comes to community empowerment, they may serve as the gatekeepers and catalysts for the change that is both desired and needed.

Knowledge needs to be more than the facts but phronesis *(Greek[1]), which is the ability to walk the talk—factual and experiential and emotional knowledge.*

There are many levels of leadership within the church in addition to the clergy, people who are often key to the provision of many of the services and ministries of the church. It is vital that they, too, understand the rationale for mainstreaming competence and the process involved. They may need to be supported, have their capacity built, and be accompanied in the process.

Staff Retreat Process

> Do not start with your gifts or "capacities" but with what God is calling you to do and to be. —*Anonymous*

In preparation for mainstreaming, a suggested exercise is to hold a retreat[2] for the leadership of all departments of the church. The following are areas for reflection, commitment, and competence in order to make a significant difference in the way we respond, why we respond, how we respond, and what the desired outcome to our response ultimately is. The retreat process can involve:

- Reflections on who we are as church and how we understand or relate to issues of HIV and AIDS.
- HIV and AIDS information sessions; encounters with persons living with HIV and hearing their testimonies; DVDs/videos that throw fresh light onto new topics or challenge current understandings or preconceptions, such as (a) explanations of the "SAVE" message (which replaces the ABC acronym),[3] (b) multiple challenges faced by HIV-positive children and adolescents, (c) the scourge of and silence surrounding gender-based violence, or (d) challenges of alternative sexual orientation.
- Reflections and dialogue on inner competence for inner transformation and empowerment[4] through the acknowledgment of attitudes and the recognition of risks and vulnerabilities of ourselves and of our church.
- Opportunity to experience pre-testing counselling and to undergo an HIV test.
- Developing understanding of what HIV competence is in terms of: knowledge, theological and technical competence, social relevance and inclusiveness, networking and collaboration, advocacy, assessment, and use of all available resources.
- Exploring the church's HIV and AIDS policy (see 5.4, Int, Ms. 4A above).
- Discussing awareness of HIV within the workplace, the church as an employer, confidentiality issues, and how to deal with HIV in the workplace (the workplace policy; see 5.4, Int, Ms. 4A above).

- Internal discussions on the value, process, and implications of HIV main-streaming, as such a process will require commitment from those involved at every level.
- Visiting another church/institution already actively involved in developing HIV competence and mainstreaming to see, appreciate, listen, learn, and transfer knowledge and experiences.
- Introducing Contextual Bible Study methodology[5] as a useful and effective tool to confront many issues, which are often contentious, using Scripture as the source of stories and as inspiration in understanding such problems within our own day and context; for instance, the rape of Tamar (2 Samuel 13:1-22).

Summary: Hold a retreat for leadership of all departments of the church to:
- Reflect on who are we as church and how we identify with HIV and AIDS.
- Honestly acknowledge attitudes and recognize risks and vulnerabilities of ourselves and of our church.
- Consider gender issues that are fundamental to the risks and vulnerabilities.
- Discuss workplace issues.
- Build capacity in the staff to cope with and mitigate the impact of HIV.
- Discuss the value of HIV mainstreaming and the implications.
- Hear the stories and learn from the experiences of those who are most affected by HIV.

Activities to Be Undertaken by Leadership

> Plans fail for lack of counsel, but with many advisors they succeed.
> —*Proverbs 15:22*

> Spirituality has to do with critiquing the present. . . . Follow
> the example of Jesus to question, question, question authority.
> . . . The tradition is being courageous enough to ask the right
> questions along the way. The courage to question the seemingly
> unquestionable is the essence of spiritual leadership . . .
> —*Sr. Joan Chittister, OSB*[6]

Sometimes messages of HIV prevention, gender-based violence, and other important issues are lost if people do not have the necessary social education on how to effectively address these issues in one's own life and community. These messages will not help to improve the life of the individual or family, for without education that imparts essential life skills and inspires belief in one's personal power to effect circumstances, a person faced with difficult decisions will struggle to apply new information or resources in positive, life-changing ways.[7] It is for this reason that considerable effort should be put into allowing the individuals and communities to identify their issues as priorities and together the necessary skills needed are identified and appropriate plans/activities are developed to address these issues.

In order for the leaders to reach an understanding of key concerns and issues faced by congregants and the community served by the church, the following actions are recommended:

A. *Listen, learn, appreciate, investigate, and seek to understand, together with target groups:*

1. What is their vision for a church and community that are affected by HIV? What kind of response would they like to see and experience? What would they like to see the church and community look like? What might be barriers to achieving this vision?

2. Where are we now? In what ways are the various members and the community currently affected by HIV and/or AIDS? Is stigma an issue, and how open are the church and its members to those in their midst who are personally affected? What impact is it having on the members and communities?

What are some of the most pressing challenges being faced by individuals, families, and communities served by the church in this context? It is important to note that the various challenging issues and risks commonly faced by the congregants and the community served by the church may be issues that the congregants and communities may not necessarily consider to be relevant to "the church and church matters" and so they may have difficulty actually articulating them (such as domestic violence). However, if there are problems that are very real to the community members themselves, they should be noted. HIV may be the end result of many such risks. It is also likely that there will be some households that are already affected, one way or another, by the impact of HIV and or AIDS and may appreciate having the space to share their burden and concerns.

What is the knowledge of the members to the risks and where to find appropriate help? What is the vulnerability of the group to the risks?

Map the services available: Who is doing what and where and for whom?

3. What do we want to do? Prioritize the risks together: What affects or concerns them the most, particularly in relation to HIV and AIDS? What do we want to do to address those risks, concerns, and vulnerabilities?

4. What can we do?

- Identify opportunities for response and the strengths that are to be found already within the church and in the community.
- Plan together on the relevant actions to be taken, and set targets to measure change.
- Identify the skills and resource materials needed by leadership and the community to respond adequately, effectively, and appropriately to the identified priorities and concerns and build capacity in these areas.
- Identify skills and resources that the target group needs to avoid risks, to minimize vulnerabilities, and to cope with the impacts of HIV and AIDS, and build capacity, as appropriate, in these areas.
- Seek out relevant partners, allies, and colleagues to strengthen the response or fill the gap.

5. Now put the plans into action and implement the activities,

6. Measure progress according to desired targets and adapt where necessary.

7. Learn from experiences; document them for now and for the future, and share.

B. *Practical ways to address prioritized risks in sermons, liturgies, prayers, and church activities:*

Liturgy: Liturgy is worship that includes silence, contemplation, words, songs, dance, and practices that are used to communicate with God in fellowship and in solitude. It is possible to mainstream HIV into the liturgies: sermons, homilies, preaching, prayers, and support offered by the church. HIV-specific liturgies for significant events like funerals have been developed, as well as liturgies used in celebration, such as healing services and prayers for those of us living with HIV or affected by it. HIV can be addressed in sermons specifically or through the contextual relevance of the Bible readings. It is vitally important though that the language used, when referring to HIV and or AIDS, and the quality of the message is nonstigmatizing, is thought provoking and inspiring, and shows the unconditional and all-encompassing love of our Lord. Too many people have received messages equating HIV with leprosy or that it is a punishment from God and thus have been alienated at perhaps their time of greatest need. Counteract stigma and show how the church is the home for all, where all can experience the redeeming love of the Lord and the acceptance of each other. Many resources have been developed by different faiths for this purpose.[8] "Talk to the congregation about the spiritual dimensions of human sexuality and about the need to protect others form harm, including protecting young people who may be subject to incest, sexual abuse, exploitation or violence."[9]

People living with HIV: Lead by example by visiting and ministering to those living with or affected by HIV in your church, and by involving people living with HIV in the life of the church.[10] They can be valuable resource people in the parish response to HIV as they have the most experience of the virus in their daily lives and are the most aware of what helps and what hinders them in the challenge of living positively with the virus. Invite people who are living with the virus to share their stories with the congregation. Call for understanding and protection of people living with HIV and their families and acceptance. Through sensitive teaching and preaching and exercising pastoral care, religious leaders can influence the congregation's attitude toward those most affected, allowing them to live more meaningful and dignified lives.

Information: Ensure publications, periodicals, newsletters, and the like, specifically addressing HIV issues, are made available or can be easily accessed. Develop or provide the necessary educational resources for young people on issues of prevention and include input from people living with HIV. Make use of the many resources freely available from the World Council of Churches, Ecumenical Advocacy Alliance, and others (see appendix).

Contextual Bible Study[11] is a useful and effective tool to confront many of the more sensitive and contentious issues. The methodology involves a fresh way of rereading familiar passages as well as lesser-known passages from the Bible, understanding the context in which the events took place and seeking to find the relevance of the event for the readers today, especially considering the same passages "through the eyes of HIV." It is a stimulating way to increase understanding of issues faced by persons living with or affected by HIV. It also affords opportunity to discuss the more difficult and contentious issues, such as rape, incest, gender-based violence, power relationships, discrimination, and exclusion by using the Bible as the textbook providing the key stories. This methodology can be encouraged in church, group, or home Bible studies to promote a new way of viewing relationships between men and women. It reinforces the need for zero tolerance of violence and upholds the value that the Lord places on women and children. It provides a platform for each participant, encouraging communication that is honest, positive, affirming, and life giving.

Safe spaces: Create "safe spaces" in the church, which are sacred spaces where critical issues that are not often openly discussed can be dealt with, such as stigma associated with disease, HIV, gender-based violence, abuse within intimate relationships, human sexuality, and sexual relationships. These important subjects are rooted in the ethical discernment, beliefs, and moral choices of individuals and society and contribute to behavioural and societal responses. These issues can be divisive for faith communities, so openness and a nonprescriptive approach are vital to enable positive transformation.[12]

HIV-positive parents may need counselling and support to help them talk to their children about their illness. Churches, in collaboration with organizations for people living with HIV, are able to broach these subjects, providing technical expertise to ensure that wishes are respected and to accompany the person through these events. Children may need help and spiritual guidance to understand and accept the illness of their parents.

In addition, parents may need help and support at the appropriate time to explain and disclose to their HIV-positive children their serostatus and the implications it has for them at school, on the sports field, if injured, in relationships, and in coming to terms with their sexuality. Again, such children will need accompaniment and understanding, especially as they work through the "Why me?" questions, anger, and grief.

Advocacy: The church has a prophetic role and could raise a voice to challenge governments, health-care systems, and social-service systems to uphold the rights of people, particularly those living with HIV, orphans, vulnerable children, and others negatively affected by HIV. Advocate for social justice and the end to discriminatory practices, especially gender-related practices, and speak against violence in any form. Advocate for universal access to lead by example and encourage testing for HIV: "Know your status!"

Example: Extract from World AIDS Day service in the Anglican Church, Cape Town, South Africa, 2009

Commitment *(we say together):*

I commit myself to work for an AIDS-free future. I know that change starts with me.

I recognize that sexuality is a sacred gift from God. I commit myself to treat my body and my partner as a temple of the Holy Spirit. I recognize that HIV is mainly spread through unsafe sex and I commit myself to protect myself and those I love.

I commit myself to be a role model to others in the community and I commit myself to support those made vulnerable to HIV through poverty, age, or gender imbalance.

I know that HIV is a medical condition, and that the body of Christ has HIV-positive members. I commit myself to combat discrimination in any form.

I recognize that HIV is fuelled by gender-based violence and I commit myself to challenge attitudes and beliefs that increase vulnerability of women.

I recognize the importance of testing and commit myself to knowing my status.

I recognize that there are many people who are living with HIV who need support, and I commit myself to reach out in practical ways to those in need.

I know that God has a special place in His heart for orphans, and I commit myself to do my part in their lives.

I commit myself to work for an AIDS-free future.

The change starts with me.

Benchmarks on Competence

These benchmarks were developed as a self-assessment and peer evaluation tool to help institutions and churches chart progress or lack of it. They were compiled during the development of *Beacons of Hope* and have similar relevance here. The appropriate benchmarks will be found at the conclusion of each section as a guideline and are not expected to be prescriptive.

Homilies/Preaching: The spoken word and the writing we commit on paper in the place of worship and in the context of worship, as leaders, clergy, and laity.

- How often do we hear HIV being addressed in sermons (never, once, or more events)?
- What is the quality of the message (stigmatizing, poor, good, inspiring/thought-provoking)?
- Are our leaders knowledgeable and trained on the issue (no, adequate, good level)?
- Have there been specific publications/periodicals/newsletters addressing HIV (none, one, two, more than three)?
- Is the issue addressed in other publications/periodicals/newsletters (none, one, two, three, four, or more)?

Liturgy: Worship that includes silence, contemplation, words, songs, dances, and practices that are used to communicate with God in fellowship and in solitude.

- Do we have HIV-specific liturgies for funerals, marriages, confirmation (no, yes)?
- Have our routine liturgies incorporated and addressed HIV (no, yes)?
- Do we celebrate healing services/liturgies (no, yes)?
- Do we say special prayers for those of us who are living with HIV and affected by it (no, yes)?
- Do we include testimonies from HIV-positive people (no, yes)?

Faith formation and moral education: The formation that helps us to incorpo-rate Christian values into our daily lives. Have we incorporated HIV (in the form of change in curriculum, addition of workshops and seminars, and so forth) in our:

- Sunday schools?
- Youth groups?
- Women's fellowships?
- Men's fellowships?
- For the whole congregation?

These are guidelines and many other checkpoints could be added.

Specific Areas in the Life and Ministry of the Church for Mainstreaming

Matthew 25:35-36 Contextualized
- I was hungry for education, training and skills and you gave me the education, the training and the skills needed to find something to eat, to excel in and to celebrate;
- I was thirsty for information, self-empowerment and self-actualization—you gave all that to me and quenched my soul's thirst;
- I was a stranger in a world of work, employable skills, information technology, societal advancement and fulfilled dreams—you invited me in;
- I was educationally, socially, culturally and politically at risk: naked, exposed and vulnerable to violence, exploitation and humiliation based on my age, gender, religious creed, political persuasion, colour of my skin, economic status, sexuality and geographical location; you clothed me with human dignity, political justice, social freedom, spiritual accompaniment and economic emancipation;
- I was sick and dying from preventable, treatable and controllable infections and illnesses related to and beyond HIV and AIDS; you nursed me, supported me and brought me back to my feet, my job and to my health and well-being;
- I was in a strong-walled prison of stigma, shame, denial, discrimination, humiliation and exclusion—bowed down with high mountains of despair, huge rivers of self and societal hate and deep valleys of hopelessness; you visited me there, entered my pain and released my chains. —*Canon Dr. Gideon Baguma Byamugisha*[1]

8.1 Children in Church: The Child in the Midst
Throughout Scripture, children play a significant and sometimes central role in God's plan for God's people whether it was the Hebrew baby Moses in the basket in the Egyptian bulrushes; the child Samuel who was the answer to

Hannah's heartfelt prayer and who later became the first judge of Israel; young Joseph, the favoured son sold as a slave into Egypt by his brothers; the shepherd boy David who stood against the Philistine giant and delivered Israel; and many, many more such examples. Indeed, Jesus himself took on our humanity and was born as a vulnerable child in a simple manager: ". . . and a little child shall lead them" (Isa. 11:6).

God also uses the analogy of children and of being a Father to them when referring to God's people and the love, care, and guidance God offers them so unconditionally.

In Matthew's Gospel (Chapter 18, 1-5) Jesus made a significant gesture when he took a little child (not a woman, poor man or a Gentile), and placed him in the middle of His disciples as a key to understanding the kingdom of Heaven and the very heart of His calling and mission:

> "He called a little child and had him stand among them. And he said: "I tell you the truth, unless you change and become like little children, you will never enter the kingdom of heaven. Therefore, whoever humbles himself like this child is the greatest in the kingdom of heaven. And whoever welcomes a little child like this in my name welcomes me."

God chose to place a child in the middle of human history. The immediate reaction was that this divine child was placed in a manger because there was no room for Him in the inn. Perhaps even today we do not make room for Him, in the form of a child, in our theology, biblical studies, worship and pastoral work.[2]

For several hundreds of years, children have been the object of mission and churches have recognized the need to introduce children to Christian teachings from an early age and to respond to their immediate perceived needs. Is this sufficient today? Are we missing something important? Can we come to understand more of the heart of God through our interactions with children? Increasingly, the idea of "a theology of children" is a growing phenomenon, leading us to explore and reflect on many fundamental theological issues of the human condition from a different perspective.

Children today face so many challenges. Families may be fractured or simply nonexistent, affecting children's physical and psychological well-being. Parental love and supervision may be missing. Role models may be faulty or absent. The family setting where one would expect nurturing and growth to take place in a secure environment may not be there or have some weak or inappropriate substitute. It is no longer a safe world for children and there is plenty of evidence of neglect, exploitation, and abuse of children in homes and even within the church and church-run institutions. Such places do not necessarily provide a safe space for children; indeed, children are very much sinned against.

We do not always have answers for the suffering of children and we may fail in our efforts to comfort. But try we must. We must seek to understand their vulnerabilities, both internally and externally, and what children are facing in their day-to-day life and experiences. Where appropriate, we need to identify and seek to address the external stressors on their households and individual lives as well as provide adequate psychosocial support to build on their resilience to cope, and perhaps most of all, making sure they do not feel alone in their circumstances.

> The role of churches in relation to children is to promote a society in which every child is valued and all children have the opportunity 'to grow up as competent and confident learners and communicators, healthy in mind, body, and spirit, secure in their sense of belonging and in the knowledge that they make a valued contribution to the society.'
>
> This is a theological imperative. As the Body of Christ, and the Family of God in the world, the church's responsibility for children is sealed in such concepts as baptism, the promise of blessing, and the gift of creation. As God has nurtured the church, so too the church communities are called to provide for children, and to nurture them in the love of God.
>
> The church is in a unique position to proclaim and execute God's blessing and justice for children. Charged with a theological imperative and grounded with a biblical mandate, the church is the voice of the voiceless as it calls a people and a nation to care for children within the church and beyond.[3]

Many churches have or are in the process of developing mandatory child protection policies for the church, with clearly defined procedures to be undertaken in the event of any breech or perceived breech of protocol in relating to children in the church.

> Good children do not just happen. They are the result of careful cultivation. —*Isaiah 54:13, paraphrase*

In addition to the identified challenges faced by children today, there are the added challenges of HIV, whether as an infection ravaging their bodies or as collateral damage resulting from the impact of HIV and AIDS on their primary caregivers and homes.

Every year 390,000 children are born with HIV. HIV transmission can be prevented, and every child can be born free of HIV. A considerable amount of commitment is needed to change this situation and stigma and discrimination needs to be eradicated in this area. While some mothers seek treatment for their own condition, there are many who do not take their HIV-positive child for treatment as it will expose their own serostatus, both to health-facility staff and to others who might see the child's medication or treatment cards, who then make stigmatizing assumptions.

Children who are born HIV-positive, or who have an HIV-positive parent or caregiver, may need help and spiritual guidance to understand, accept, and cope with their own emotions. Church leadership should have the knowledge of who is appropriately trained, and could be called upon, to accompany the children and parents/caregivers as required.

> The test of the morality of a society is what it does for its children.
> —*Dietrich Bonhoeffer*

Protection Protocols

It is well known that most Sunday school and confirmation teachers and church youth-club workers are volunteers in the church who feel called to serve in this capacity. Some are remunerated for their time given. Whatever the situation, though such willingness and service is to be applauded, the church has a real responsibility for the children who are entrusted into its care and for their appropriate instruction. There is need for a clear protocol to be in place for those working with children and young people. This serves to protect beneficiaries, staff, and the church and provide guidelines on procedures to be followed in the event of any form of breach to this protocol, perceived or otherwise. All persons wishing to offer services within the church, whether as paid employees or as volunteers, need to be vetted by the church authorities to establish information on their background, motivation for such work, their knowledge and understanding of the issues involved and to ensure there is a adherence to church protocol. Mechanisms need to be in place to prevent inappropriate adult-child engagement that may lead to situations of abuse or accusations of abuse. Prevention is better than cure.

Example: Child-Friendly Church, Viva Network

The Child-Friendly Church[4] is a strategy to empower local churches to transform their local congregations and communities in favour of children. The programme has been successfully piloted across Eastern and Central Africa and is continuing in Tanzania, Kenya, South Africa, and Uganda.

How it works: church leaders complete a survey based on the eight aims of Child-Friendly Churches to identify the key development areas for their church community. Churches are given the Child-Friendly resource pack and can then receive interactive training on any or all of the eight key areas.

The Eight Aims of Child-Friendly Churches

1. *There is a vision for children's work in the church*. Churches are encouraged to empathize with God's heart for children and understand why the nurture of children is the particular responsibility of the church.
2. *Training of workers and child protection is in place and is being implemented*. Churches are trained in child-protection issues and taken through the step-by-step development and implementation of a practical child-protection policy.
3. *The church building offers a safe environment*. Churches are equipped to conduct risk assessments, including health and safety, first aid, accidents, and emergencies. They are then taught to develop corresponding policies.
4. *Nurture groups are available for children and young people*. Churches are taught the value of regular support for children through Bible teaching, peer-group nurturing, prayer, and the recognition that different children have different needs.
5. *There are opportunities for children to engage in worship in the church*. Churches are shown the importance of making main church services child friendly, as well as allowing children to plan and lead sections of services and Sunday schools.
6. *Suitable facilities for under-fives are available*. Churches understand the importance of allocating specific areas to under-fives with appropriate toys, resource,s and equipment available, as well as supporting the parents of these children well.
7. *Children and young people are involved as equal members of the church community*. Churches are encouraged to see all members of the church, young or old, as equally important and give them opportunities to express their opinions on church matters.
8. *There are outreach opportunities for and with children*. Churches see the value of community outreach which includes children in planning, implementation, and evaluation. Churches sensitize community members and duty bearers to needs of children in the community.

By helping church leaders and congregations to better understand the needs of children and involve them in their churches, the Viva network is seeing incredible growth, as increasing numbers of children come to church and bring their families with them.

Though it is a work in progress, churches are restructuring their programs and facilities to ensure that children are a priority and that they are provided with a safe and protective environment. Churches are speaking out on issues of child protection during their main services and during community gatherings which was not happening before. Churches are also becoming advocacy centers for issues of child protection in their communities. Children are being nurtured holistically in the way of the Lord as churches restructure, so as to accommodate age appropriate classes in children's church. Churches see the need to have their Sunday school teachers trained. Churches see the need for a written child protection policy and having all their staff sign up commitment forms to child protection.[5]

The next three sections outline areas in the church where we most frequently engage with children and present opportunities to *be* church to the children in our midst.

8.2 Sunday School Classes and Teachers

A training session or retreat can be held for all Sunday school teachers for the following purposes:

A. Leading guided reflections toward inner competence.

B. Raising awareness to the wider issues of HIV and AIDS, the determinants to its spread, risks, vulnerabilities, and impacts, with particular reference to the age groups attending the Sunday school classes.

C. Mapping services available within the church and as accessible referral points. Seek out partners wherever necessary.

D. Assessing risks that the children are facing, within their context, and their vulnerability not only to HIV but to other factors that in time may increase their risk to HIV. For example:

- Children may already be HIV-infected.
- They may be facing orphanhood.
- They may be living in vulnerable households.
- They are in the age group most vulnerable to other illnesses encountered with HIV-positive parents (respiratory tract infections, tuberculosis, etc.).

- They are encountering illness, grief, and loss at close quarters.
- They may be shunted around between families, or be unsupervised, unattended, exploited, or abused.
- They may encounter stigma and discrimination as a result of their own infection, their poverty status, disrupted schooling, or their home situations.

E. Identifying any relevant skills and/or training needed. These might include trainings in psychosocial support, to understand the impact of loss and grief on children and to identify other situations that may require some form of intervention or additional support. A withdrawn child or a highly disruptive child may in fact be reacting to difficult home situations they are facing and may require particularly sensitive handling.

F. Training teachers on participatory methods with children of different age groups to assess, with the children, their knowledge and understanding of the environment in which they may be growing up and their risks and vulnerabilities.

G. Guiding teachers on how to identify, with the children, the priority issues they are facing (which may represent risk factors or vulnerability factors) and their current coping mechanisms.

H. Designing or redesigning programmes to incorporate activities, Bible studies, discussions, films, and role plays to address the risks, vulnerabilities, and ways of mitigating impact. The Bible is full of relationship stories and lived experiences of people, demonstrating virtually every possible event likely to be encountered by most children in our Sunday schools. Using these stories contextually, they can be used as both an entrance point to issues, or as a means to discuss issues, consequences, choices, and options. There is room for some specific material development where such resources are lacking.

I. Incorporating life skills in all sessions: value systems, affirmation, encouragement, role models, and assertiveness as protection.

J. Making teachers aware of critical services that can be accessed for guidance or intervention if this becomes necessary. Children need to know they are not alone with their problems. God is with them, but so are we.

K. Listening to children's voices, which need to be heard: we hear their voices as the voice of the society.

The above process could equally be utilized by all teachers in church schools, not just Sunday school teachers.

8.3 Confirmation Classes

The word *confirmation* means strengthening or deepening one's relationship with God and it is a sacrament, ritual, or rite of passage practiced by several Christian denominations. Thus confirmation-class teachers will need to be properly "accredited" by the church for this role, in line with procedures for *any* person wishing to work with youth in the church and in accordance with established protocols.

Confirmation classes represent an opportunity for (principally) young people to understand the implications of the promises made on their behalf at baptism and to choose to ratify that act. It is an opportunity to review their relationship to God and to others: Where are they in terms of "I believe in God"? Is God's sovereignty over their life invited and accepted? These are life-changing and affirming choices. At this particular age, young people need to evolve from a social Sunday occasion to an inner transformation that applies to every day of the week, both for now and for the future.

Confirmation candidates attend a series of special classes to learn about the sacraments, their faith, and Christian responsibilities. A bishop usually conducts the service. At one time candidates were required to learn a series of questions and answers as the catechism. Today's classes are more comprehensive and the particular needs of candidates are considered. It is an opportunity to ensure that the candidates are helped to view the relevance and affirmation of their faith in relation to the realities they face, particularly in a world of HIV and its challenges for young people.

Young people in this age group have their own challenges and are at a sensitive age in terms of the need for identity and peer acceptance. Some of the risks they face include:

- Lack of knowledge on risks to HIV issues and lack of places to find out information from an informed nonjudgmental adult.
- Misinformation on sex, sexuality, and reproductive health issues. In the absence of youth-friendly places where youth feel secure to question and to access scientifically correct information, they most frequently turn to their (sometimes equally uninformed) peers or to the wider Internet, with its own inherent dangers.
- Exposure to harmful and confusing media messages and norms.
- Temptations to experiment with drugs, alcohol, and sex.
- Peer pressure.
- Risk-taking behaviour as part of the "macho image."
- Adolescent hormonal challenges, coupled with lack of communication skills with parents and other figures of authority, leading to a tendency toward rebellion.
- Absence of the presence of either the father or mother, for whatever reason, creating different family dynamics and challenges for all concerned.

- Possible and frequent lack of protective assertive skills when faced with exploitation or the risk of abuse.
- Not knowing whom to turn to for help, advice, comfort, encouragement, or help in life-challenging situations.

In order to be aware of the challenges that HIV and AIDS are presenting to young people, teachers working with youth may well benefit from a specific HIV-focused retreat or similar empowering process of:

A. Leading guided reflections toward inner competence.

B. Providing HIV and AIDS information sessions and encounters with HIV-positive people or youth.

C. Building understanding of the wider issues on HIV and AIDS, the determinants to spread, risks, vulnerabilities, and impacts, with particular reference to the age groups attending the confirmation classes.

D. Mapping the services available within the church and as accessible referral points. Seek out partners wherever necessary.

E. Assessing the risks that the young people are facing and their vulnerability.

F. Identifying any relevant skills and/or training needed. These might include trainings to improve understanding of the impact of HIV and AIDS on youth (especially those who have been infected since childhood), stigma, disclosure, loss and grief, psychosocial support, and empowerment. As was noted regarding Sunday school classes, withdrawn or disruptive behaviour, such as being the class clown, may be symptomatic of underlying unresolved issues that require help and sensitive handling, not punishment.

G. Providing training on participatory methods with young people, of different relevant age groups, to assess their knowledge and understanding of their environment and their risks and vulnerabilities.

Within the confirmation class:

1. *Vision*: Give them the space to share what would be their vision for their church and community in their current context, and in an era of HIV and AIDS. What would make a significant difference in their lives? How could this vision be achieved and how can their faith help them? What are the opportunities and strengths within the church and within themselves to make this possible?

2. Dialogue with youth as to where they consider themselves to be now, in relation to their vision:

- Ask them, What would be barriers to achieving this vision? As they are usually at the age of adolescence, do they have access to correct information on sexual and reproductive health to help them understand the physical and emotional changes their bodies are going through and the responsibilities these changes bring? What is their understanding and experiences of HIV and AIDS? Are they aware of the key drivers of the epidemic, transmission, and prevention of infection with HIV?

- Identify, together with the young people, the key issues they are facing (which may represent risk factors or vulnerability factors) and their current coping mechanisms.
- Help them identify risks and vulnerabilities they are experiencing within their context or communities

3. What do they *want* to do? Discuss this with them so that the overall vision is jointly realized.

4. What *can* we do?

- Prioritize the most pressing or threatening issues and agree to address at least three of them within the context of the confirmation classes as life issues.
- Help youth to identify their own personal problems, consider the consequences, examine options and choices, make careful decisions, and make changes where appropriate and necessary. Help them acknowledge the value of their conscience and to have the courage to stand for what is right, even if it not the most popular course of action. This is a process of true empowerment.
- Provide safe spaces for dialogue and sharing and questioning.
- Point them to places where they can receive the necessary information, help, or support when such services are unavailable at home or in the church.
- Integrate life-skills training in all sessions as well as value systems, affirmation, encouragement, role models, rights and responsibilities, and assertiveness as protection.
- Design or redesign programmes to integrate activities, Bible studies, discussions, films, role plays to address the risks and vulnerabilities that youth are facing today, especially in relation to HIV infection, and ways of mitigating impact. Introducing youth to Contextual Bible Study methodology is an empowering tool to help them understand relevant life skills within a common context. The Bible is full of relationship stories and lived experiences of people demonstrating virtually every possible event likely to be encountered by most youth. Using the biblical stories and events contextually can present opportunities to discuss issues that are often avoided yet are burning topics for youth.

5. Encourage youth to identify what *they* can contribute to the church.

6. Encourage young people to support each other and to share their experiences for mutual benefit and spiritual growth.[6]

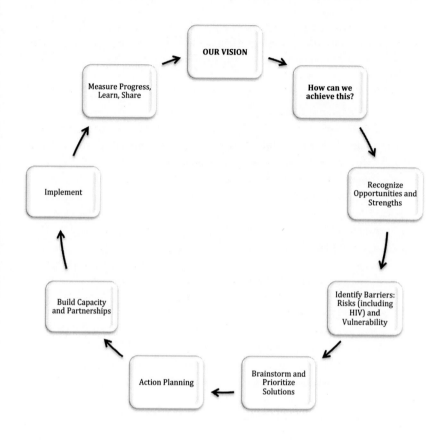

8.4 Youth Work in the Church, Church Clubs, Schools, and the Surrounding Community

Youth are the population group most affected by HIV. It is within this group that one identifies whether or not HIV is coming under control in a country. In many parishes young people, in the age bracket of 15–35 years, constitute a major percentage of the congregation.[7] Yet, demographically, they are the most unrepresented and neglected when it comes to proactive programmes to address the risks of HIV. Several studies have shown that in many African countries young people are denied their rights to education on sexual reproductive health and risky behaviours. They live in communities without adequate sources of information, means, tools, or services for protection. In both churches and health centers, there is a lack of or inadequate youth-friendly services. Frequently the youth are not consulted on the issues facing them, nor are they actively involved in the design and implementations of programmes ostensibly for them. As Paula Clifford writes,

> Bound up with this is the whole question of sex education for young people. Many church groups have argued that this also leads to promiscuity. However, research indicates that this is far from being the case. The evidence shows that sexual health and HIV education does not lower the age of sexual debut, nor does it increase sexual activity or the number of sexual partners [Mary Garvey]. Sometimes the opposite has been found to be the case, with the age of sexual debut delayed and activity reduced. In any case, the failure of parents, schools and churches to talk about sexual matters to the children in their care, is dangerously irresponsible in the face of the HIV epidemic. Embarrassment, shame or a tradition of not talking about sex until a young person is on the verge of marriage, all ensure that children and young people remain vulnerable to HIV. As the Archbishop of Cape Town has put it:
>
> > At the very point in their lives when God has given them all the physical means to love, our young people are, at times, abandoned by parents, society and the church and left to learn by themselves the life skills which sexual relationships require. In a world beset by the devastating HIV pandemic, we are leaving our young people, the flower of our church and our society, to wither and die through ignorance, the absence of open, honest and compassionate sharing of vital information, our embarrassed silence and resistance to reality.[8]

Strategically and deliberately investing in the well-being of young people can result in powerful positive individual and social change. There are vast numbers of educational facilities owned and run by the faith community. While HIV and AIDS issues can and should be mainstreamed into the life and curricula of schools, there is also nonformal space within all schools. This space can be exploited so that young people learn compassion, respect, nonstigmatizing or judgmental attitudes, and how to be active members of their community. It is also a place where accurate information on HIV and its prevention can be accessed. Counselling services can be offered within the schools, and teachers could be trained in psychosocial support and counselling skills. For example: a child/youth who is disruptive in class frequently is routinely punished but his or her behaviour may be a reaction to serious stresses that the child is facing in the home environment. Teachers who have not been sensitized may not consider this when responding and hence may aggravate the situation, and stigma, for the child concerned. Humanitarian services also need to view the services through the lens of HIV such as ensuring there are adequate ablution facilities and separate toilets for girls and boys.

There are opportunities to promote youth-driven clubs such as "Stop the Silence Clubs," "Stop AIDS," "Youth against AIDS," and the like. It is also an ideal opportunity to unpack the gender scripting under which youth are raised that may make them more vulnerable to HIV infection. Boys need to have opportunity to critically explore masculinities that promote the macho image whereby they are encouraged to be dominant in relationships and sexual decisions. To have multiple relationships is seen as a sign of manhood and power. Girls and women, on the other hand, are raised to be subservient and deferential to boys and men, with little control over decision making in their lives. Both sexes are thus made more vulnerable in the era of HIV.

Effective programs must be driven by the vision and perceptions of youth and increasingly adopt an *assets-based* and a *solutions-based* approach to youth development instead of a *problem-focused* one.[9]

8.4.1 Activities with Youth Leaders

Religious leaders need to build their own capacities to engage with youth. As discussed previously, all persons wishing to offer services within the church, whether as paid employees or as volunteers, need to be vetted by the church authorities to establish motivation, understanding of the issues involved, and a clear protocol to protect beneficiaries, staff, and the church; this is particularly important in areas of work with young people.

At the same time, all those working with young people and children should feel valued and receive the appropriate training and support they need. Youth leaders should, first and foremost, attend a retreat or training that covers the following basics:

A. Leading guided reflections toward inner competence.

B. Building understanding of the wider issues on HIV and AIDS, the determinants to its spread, risks, vulnerabilities, and impacts, with particular reference to the age groups attending the youth club.

C. Mapping the services available within the church and at accessible referral points, which youth may need. Youth leaders should not feel burdened with problems presented by youth, which may be outside of the scope, ability, or experience of the youth leaders. Appropriate referral is the most sensible and safest option. Seek out partners wherever necessary.

D. Assessing the identified and known risks that youth are facing and their vulnerability within their environments and communities.

E. Identifying any relevant skills and/or training needed. These might include trainings to understand the impact of HIV and AIDS on youth, especially those who have been infected since childhood, stigma, disclosure, loss and grief, psychosocial support, and empowerment. Both a withdrawn young person and a highly disruptive youth may be suffering from the same root causes to their problem and require equally sensitive handling.

F. Providing training on participatory methods with young people, of different relevant age groups, to assess their knowledge and understanding of their environment and their risks and vulnerabilities.

G. Seeking out relevant partners, allies, and colleagues. Establish strategic relationships with referral systems (e.g., abuse survivors, counselling and testing centers, counselling services, support groups, etc.). Provide exposure to programmes in other churches and centers from which there is much to learn and share best practices.

8.4.2. Activities with the Youth

While there are similarities in the activities with young people in confirmation classes and with all the other youth, these two categories have been separated within this document as the departments are often separate within the church even though there is obviously overlap and more age-specific activities within the two departments. The following represent suggested ways of working with youth:

1. *Vision*: Encourage youth, including those living with the virus or affected by it, to share their concerns and hopes, encouraging open discussion of values, sexual integrity, and healthy relationships. What is their vision of a preferred future, their *dream* for the future? What would they like to see in their own life, in their church and in their community in the future?

How could this vision be achieved? What opportunities are there for such a vision to become a reality? What strengths are already there that can be drawn upon, both from within the youth themselves and from the surrounding support networks of families, friends, the church, and others?

2. Where are we *now*? What is the current situation and what barriers are there to achieving this goal? What priority issues are youth facing? What might pose risks? What risks might ultimately render youth vulnerable to HIV and the impact of AIDS? How much knowledge exists in the group on HIV and what are their personal experiences, attitudes, and understandings of HIV and where to source the necessary information and support?

a. *Examples of risks/concerns faced by youth.*
- Lack of accurate up-to-date information on issues of sex and sexuality, HIV risks, prevention of HIV, and how to mitigate impact
- Lack of sources of information—safe places from which to access credible, nonjudgmental information
- Dysfunctional families; divorce of parents and alternative caregivers; and lack of family guidance, love, and emotional support
- Heavy expectations from teachers and family alike to achieve, leading to substantial stress, with few or no coping strategies
- Difficulties balancing demands of home, of school, of sport, of income-generating activities because of financial constraints and peer pressure
- Peer pressure, sexual coercion, and lack of ability to deal with this
- Exposure to exploitative and confusing media messages
- Exposure to and temptation of substance abuse and experimental sex
- Domestic violence
- Abuse
- Bullying at school
- Unemployment and lack of self-esteem
- Transactional sex offers
- Financial pressures
- Already HIV-positive and lacking knowledge and skills on disclosure and how to have normal relationships like their peers without discrimination or ostracism

b. *Vulnerability of youth within their context.*
- Unsupervised youth
- Orphans
- Lack of support structures
- Risky environment, such as prevalent beer halls
- Poverty, which influences choices
- Alcohol excess at home
- Sexual violence—often hidden and unreported
- Other—to be identified together with youth

c. *Knowledge of the youth about risks and where to find information and/or help.* Explore these areas with the youth. Do not assume they have all the knowledge on risks or appropriate information on their rights and where to access the necessary support or help. Sometimes young people may ask difficult questions—it is vital that the youth leader be honest if the answers are not known and also willing to find out. Never attempt to deceive young people or trust may be damaged.

d. *Identify whether or not youth have the necessary skills and ability to deal with the risks.*

- Build ability to identify issues and thus risks
- Reduce risks and address issues at stake
- Prevent issues from becoming risks, for instance, through life-skills training, assertiveness, support structures, "shoulder to cry on," legal protection and safe spaces
- Mitigate against impact
- Receive support if impact is felt
- Build knowledge of where to find support if needed

3. What do we *want* to do? Prioritize the risks based on risk assessment and identified needs. Identify at least three and agree to work on them within the youth club.

4. What *can* we do?

- *Map the services available.* Youth are naturals with computers and other modern electronic devices. They have talents, enthusiasm, and creativity. They can be an invaluable resource as data collectors and the process of data collection is an excellent awareness tool. Point them to places where they can receive the necessary information, help, or support in the absence of there being such services available at home or in the church.
- *Ensure information resources are readily available.* Create safe spaces where dialogue can take place and accurate, up-to-date, and nonjudgmental information is readily available.
- *Identify skills and resource materials* needed by youth to deal with identified risks.
- *Design or redesign programmes to integrate activities*: Bible studies, discussions, exposure visits to other programmes, films, and role plays to address the risks, vulnerabilities, and ways of mitigating impact. The Bible is full of relationship stories and lived experiences of people demonstrating virtually every possible event likely to be encountered by most youth. Careful use of biblical stories and events contextually can present opportunities to discuss issues that are often avoided yet are burning topics for youth.
- *Engage young people in peer-to-peer support groups and prevention clubs* in hard-hit communities. Encourage the participation of young people in developing and running religious and community programmes that inform other young people about HIV prevention and develop necessary life and self-assertiveness skills to cope with negative peer pressures and ensure there is understanding about the rights of youth balanced with the responsibilities of youth in society. Use the forum to dialogue on gender scripting roles and the value of transformative masculinity.

- *Incorporate life-skills training in all sessions* as well as value systems, affirmation, encouragement, role models, rights and responsibilities, and assertiveness as protection. Help youth to identify their problems, consider the consequences, examine options and choices, and make careful decisions.

5. *Implement and measure progress according to agreed targets.* Youth need to also be encouraged to identify what they can contribute to the church. Involving them in care and support programmes can be mutually beneficial as they see and experience firsthand the implications of HIV. Young people's skills with computers and other means of information technology are underutilized in churches, as youth can be excellent data collectors and conduits for valuable information dissemination to wider audiences. Actively involving young people in their own programmes and eliciting their assistance in the other HIV programmes of the church is far more effective and motivating for them to take seriously the issues at stake than by just providing them with necessary information on protection against the risks of HIV.

6. Document experiences for sharing, and as a means of monitoring and evaluating what has been achieved.

Example: HIV Prevention Programme for Youth: Youth Media Literacy Project of the Anglican Church, Cape Town, South Africa

Background: In 2005, the HIV and AIDS programme of the Anglican Church in the Diocese of Cape Town, South Africa, conducted research into the sexual activity of Anglican Youth. Results indicated high levels of sexual activity (40 percent male, 21 percent female) amongst teenagers.[10] Based on the research, an HIV-prevention programme of peer education called "Agents of Change" was developed and piloted and has been operating since 2006 in three Dioceses of the Western Cape.

The Goal: To improve young people's life skills, assist them in improving their ability to connect their values and beliefs with their everyday practices, and aim to create a critical mass of young people exerting "positive" peer pressure to reduce risky sexual activity and thus ultimately contribute to turning the HIV and AIDS tide.

Approach: The programme aims to increase the effectiveness of the church in addressing the sexuality of young people. At a three-day training camp, peer educators and facilitators are trained in presentation skills to present 20 sessions of a life-skills training to young people of their church and their community. These are interactive sessions using a lot of ice breakers, skits, drama, and debates. The peer educators are mentored and supported by their youth leaders who are trained as facilitators.

Content: The programme aims to increase abstinence and reduce the incidence of risky sexual behaviour through the following methods:

- *By building self-efficacy and self-esteem amongst the youth.* The programme recognizes that behaviour change does not come about by information but, rather, through inspiration and affirmation. By being chosen as peer educators, the young people are inspired to make a difference in their communities and to become role models.
- *By creating positive peer pressure.* It is very hard for young people as individuals to say no to sexual activity if their friends are all sexually active. This programme aims to build positive peer pressure so that young people can encourage one another. The peer educators are encouraged to "live the message as well as give the message" so that they can become role models to their peers.
- *By developing a critical consciousness about sexual health.* Gender norms and high levels of sexual coercion put young women at high risk of infection. This programme, through participatory education, enables the young people to gain a critical consciousness regarding the gender norms of society. They are taught to understand and challenge "rape-supportive myths" such as the belief that "Girls who say no mean yes," or dressing in a "sexy" way means they are asking for sex. Critical consciousness is also developed through encouraging media literacy.

The Influence of Mass Media: Whereas 50 years ago, a teenager's family, friends, school, and church were probably the primary influences on his or her attitudes, values, and beliefs about sexuality, today's teens have access to a fifth powerful influence: mass media.[11]

A primary challenge of teenagers is self-definition. Many teens draw heavily from media images as they wrestle with who they are and where they fit in the world. When they find people or situations that resonate with their lives, they pay attention. Social cognitive theory suggests that adolescents learn and model much from the media. At this stage of their lives they are developing their identities, and through the influence of the media they learn socially acceptable ways to engage in intimate relationships.[12] Modeling may take place through a conscious copying of media roles or behaviours. It may also take place through a subconscious embodiment of the values embedded in the media content. The media are important because of the high proportion of time that young people spend under media influence, through movies, music, the Internet, and advertising. The media have the potential to encourage the acceptance of casual sex and multiple partners, as well as sexualizing women and girls and normalizing sexual coercion and violence.

> The message from advertisers and the mass media to girls (as eventual women) is they should always be sexually available, always have sex on their minds, be willing to be dominated and even sexually aggressed against and they will be gazed on as sexual objects.[13]

The influence of the media is especially problematic when it happens to youth. Developing a sense of oneself as a sexual being is an important task of adolescence. Just at the time when girls begin to construct their identity, they are more likely to suffer losses in self-esteem, and perceived physical attractiveness is closely linked to self-esteem. Diminishing self-esteem in early adolescence may make girls particularly vulnerable to cultural messages that promise popularity, love and social acceptance through the right "sexy" look.[14]

Media Literacy: Given the importance of the influence of media on young people, one of the goals of the Agents of Change programme is to increase media literacy: an important skill in reading different types of advertisements, movies, and music. Young people are taught to look at advertisements and to ask: What they are trying to sell, and how they are trying to sell it? What messages are being given? Do we agree with them or disagree? Media-literacy sessions enable young people to identify the underlying messages of lyrics or advertising and to decide for themselves whether that message is one that they identify with or reject. This can help them to avoid an unconscious acceptance and modelling of negative media messages.

Impact of the Programme: The Agents of Change programme was evaluated over a two-year period by using a quasi-experimental study comparing intervention churches with control churches (those which were not running the programme). The programme had a statistically significant impact on raising the age of sexual debut for those not yet sexually active, and increasing use of condoms amongst those who were sexually active.

8.4.4 Youth in the Community: Street Children

"Street children" are a growing reality in many countries across the world. These are children who live on the margins of society and for whom the street has either become their "permanent" home where their daily struggle is endured, or it is the place to which they drift on a daily basis for survival. There are many reasons children end up on the streets: some are runaway children who may have fled homes where domestic violence and/or abuse is common; some are separated from families in conflict or displacement; many are orphans as a consequence of AIDS or conflict or have been rejected; some have left conditions of severe poverty at home, and there are those who are sent onto the streets to earn for family members—usually in hardship. There is also a growing phenomenon of second-generation and even third-generation street children who are born to a life on the streets; such hardships are perpetuated through the generations.

Children on the streets are stigmatized, lack educational opportunities, and often have poor health and nutrition. They may be already, or become, HIV-infected. They are frequently abused, even by the police and those in authority, as they are seen as a "nuisance" and as having no rights. They are also largely "anonymous" as they have no identity records, they have little protection from anyone, and do not belong to any identifiable community—all of which increases their vulnerability hugely and limits their opportunities or access to any services, including health. Few national governments are addressing their needs and, if anything, may round them up as criminals and treat them as such. It is largely left to NGOs and faith groups to reach out to these children with a helping and compassionate hand.

While such children are ignored, avoided, rejected, violated, and often seen as victims of their situation, they are in fact resilient and tough if they can survive on their own in such a difficult environment. And even more: they, too, have dreams, hopes, and aspirations.[15] Let us not forget them when we consider the young people of society. They are the peers of our own children and are just as precious in the eyes of God.

Example: Ministry to Street Children in Antananarivo, Madagascar

Madagascar is a large island which has a lot of poverty, and consequently street children are many. Beggars are common and families may beg together. It is not uncommon to see groups of small children huddled in doorways or begging in the traffic, even with tiny babies strapped on their backs. These children may be seen at all hours of the day or night. For so many, the street is their only home.

One of the local churches, Ambavahadimitafo, has introduced a twice-weekly feeding programme for street children and vulnerable schoolchildren. Members of the church contribute the food—rice, lentils, sugar, and so forth—and take turns to prepare and serve it. The youngest children come first, in the early evening, bringing themselves from all over the city. After washing their hands, they sit in the pews and are taught a couple of songs, and hear a Bible story and a prayer. Some of them are so small they are unable to climb up onto the pews unaided. Plates of food and bread are distributed, which are consumed hungrily. While the children are eating, the volunteers circulate and are there for the children so that the children can turn to them for loving care and help. After the little ones leave, the older children come and the same procedure takes place. The church has an agreement with the police to stay away. Many of the older children survive by pick-pocketing and the police know the youths come for a meal. The church has persuaded the authorities not to harass the youth on the night(s) that they come to the church. Their outreach to the youth may be the most positive start to befriend them and hear about their circumstances, encourage them, and ultimately help them find an alternative lifestyle.

This initiative is a committed, loving response to a very marginalized and neglected sector of society, and is directly meeting a practical need. It does not seek external funding or any other support. It is a gentle quiet outreach that makes a difference to hundreds of such children.

8.5 Women's Fellowships/Guilds/Unions/Groups

Women have played a central role in the life of the Christian church since the earliest ages. Over time various groups, specifically for women, have developed in churches. Within the Anglican community they are called Mothers' Union; in the Catholic Church they are the Women's Guilds; and within all other denominations they have specific identifying names.

The role of these groups varies from denomination to denomination but at the core such women's groups support their local church with prayer, Bible studies, and social outreaches. They also support in particular the local community. Some have activities that are limited to Bible study and fundraising, others have social outreaches to women with activities such as exercise classes and other domestic and social events. Some have particular concern for the plight of women and, like the Anglican Mothers' Union, have projects that promote literacy and development, parenting, microfinance, and campaigning for gender equity and against gender-based violence, including the trafficking of women. The vision of this particular denomination's Mothers' Union is "a world where God's love is shown through loving, respectful and flourishing relationships." They seek to demonstrate the Christian faith in action by transforming communities worldwide through the nurture of the family in its many forms.

Whatever their form, women's groups in the church have a unique opportunity to engage on issues that affect all women, not only those "out there" but "those in our midst." It is an opportunity to be relevant to the issues that women are facing on a daily basis in their individual lives, in marriage, in their families, at work, and in their community. All women have dreams and, for many, life presents so many challenges and burdens that their dreams fade and are not able to flourish. Women are the backbone of society and the church can do so much to affirm them, support them, protect them, and value their immense contribution to society. This involves appreciating their dreams and visions, acknowledging their strengths, helping them find opportunities, identifying barriers and risks such as HIV, and recognizing their vulnerabilities to these risks. It means finding solutions together and planning to be able to implement effectively such solutions with the necessary training, awareness, support, and partnership.

The majority of people infected with HIV in Africa are women and they also carry the heaviest burden in terms of care. Marriage is becoming an "at-risk environment," as some 40 percent of new cases of HIV are being seen in what were previously considered "low-risk heterosexual people." Women may be afraid to discuss issues of HIV with their spouses and yet fear infection. HIV-related stigma and discrimination are found in all societies and can lead to social isolation and even loss of family support. Fear of such prejudice can cause some women to refuse HIV testing or not to return for their results. Often the greatest worry is the reaction of a male partner.[16]

Women's clubs may provide the "safe space" that they need to engage in dialogue on issues, including sensitive matters such as domestic violence, marital rape, and child abuse. They may also "provide an opportunity for HIV-positive women to meet others in the same situation, and enable women to share their experiences, fears and uncertainties in a safe, supportive and non-judgmental environment. Such groups can also support women with issues such as discrimination, sexual health awareness, sexual violence, relationships, parenting, and future options."[17]

It is also an opportunity to unpack false theology frequently taught which reinforces the oppression of women and may put them in positions of HIV risk, such as the theology promoting subservience and submission, even in abusive marital relationships. Where life skills are often given to youth to empower them in self-assertiveness, such life skills are equally important for women, especially for those who have never had the necessary training or support. Thus women's clubs in church can be a place where women may receive psychosocial support, learn necessary coping strategies, and find guidance to helpful referral and support systems.

Women's clubs can also be a useful forum in which education on antiretroviral therapy and the necessity for treatment adherence, "treatment literacy," is provided, allowing opportunity for frank discussions on the practical implications of such therapy as well as the benefits. Through a participatory process, women within their groups or clubs may be assisted to:

1. Describe what their vision or dream is for their lives, for a truly caring and supportive church, and for better communities for themselves and for their families, particularly in an era of HIV and AIDS. What would it take to achieve this vision? What strengths are there amongst the individuals and church and amongst the social networks?

2. Identify barriers to achieving this vision. What risks are there, including the risk of HIV infection? Identify principle issues of concern that pose risks to the women and ultimately that render them vulnerable to HIV and the impact of AIDS.

a. *Issues/risks faced and identified by women*:
- Unquestioning obedience to cultural norms and expectations
- Use of Scripture to oppress women
- Lack of assertiveness to voice concerns and to stand up for themselves
- Financial dependency
- Lack of negotiating skills
- Lack of communication skills between couples
- Lack of skills in conflict management
- Relationship issues and problems
- Domestic violence and abuse
- Caring for HIV-infected relatives
- Unfaithful husbands
- Discordant couples
- Dealing with stigma associated with HIV
- Substance abuse within the family

b. *Vulnerability of women within their context*. It is important to remember, especially when referring to women, that people are "made vulnerable," they are not "intrinsically vulnerable." The root cause of most violence against women is power: unequal power relationships. Often such violence is excused by culture, which may be subverted by those who maintain their status. Furthermore, though not yet universally acknowledged, marital rape is violence against women. Sexual violence is often hidden because of shame, fear, stigma, and lack of any form of guaranteed personal support should the crime be exposed. Yet there is a well-recognized close intersection between gender-based violence and HIV. Culture (and tradition) cannot and should not ever be placed above human rights.

c. *Knowledge of women about risks and where to find information and/or help*. It is often difficult for women at risk to seek help, especially if they fear their partner's reaction. Sometimes this help may be needed at short notice, such as a "safe-house" in the event of domestic violence. It is really helpful if women are made aware of where they can access support and to whom they can turn.

d. *Current coping mechanisms and skills of women to deal with risks*. Ability to:

- Identify issues and risks (of HIV infection) and vulnerability
- Reduce risks and address issues at stake
- Address prevention issues (e.g., life-skills training, assertiveness, support structures, legal protection, safe spaces)
- Mitigate against impact
- Receive support if affected

3. Dialogue on what they want to do about their situation.

4. Decide on what course of action to take and what they can do. For example:

a. *Prioritize the risks* based on risk assessment and identified needs. Identify at least three and agree to work on them within the women's club.

b. *Map the services available* such as the availability and accessibility to support groups, safe houses (places of safety to which women can go if facing domestic violence or other forms of abuse), counseling facilities, HIV testing centers, legal advice, and support agencies and places that advise on substance abuse and other similar matters. This is important as individuals may need to know where to access advice and assistance or where to refer people for such services.

c. *Identify the skills and resource materials needed* by women to deal with identified risks. For example: Members of the group might decide they need training or help in some of the following areas:

- Stress management
- Legal guidance in cases of abuse
- Taking care of oneself in order to take care of others
- Communication skills
- Conflict resolution skills
- Information on sexual reproductive health and appropriate advice
- Other identified needs

d. *Design or redesign programmes* to integrate activities, Bible studies, discussions and films, shared stories of people living with HIV or people affected by HIV who have to deal with the impacts, role-plays and dialogues to address the risks, vulnerabilities, and ways of mitigating impact. The Bible is full of relationship stories and lived experiences of people demonstrating virtually every possible event likely to be encountered by most women. Use of biblical stories and events contextually can present opportunities to discuss issues that are often avoided, particularly issues such as gender-based violence, stigma, sexuality, and others. Create safe spaces within the church where confidentiality is respected and openness can be experienced as well as a sense of solidarity and not being alone. Find strategic partners to accompany or strengthen the initiative where necessary.

5. Implement the agreed activities together.

6. Measure progress, document, and share the process with others within the church, community, and other churches to assist them also and to learn from their experiences in similar initiatives.

8.6 Men's Fellowships/Ministry/Associations/Groups

It is said that the gender gap in a church is associated with a church in decline. It is a common phenomenon that, in many countries and in many denominations, the congregations are principally composed of women and church volunteers tend to be predominantly women. Many churches have become "feminized," where women feel at home and welcomed but men may feel out of place, with limited roles in the service of the church.[18] Frequently in churches, there is very poor attendance at men's groups or fellowships. Too often, there appears to be a lack of creativity in the programmes and the role of the group tends to concentrate on fundraising. "High-achieving men" typically get fed up with churches because of the inefficiency of church meetings, unproductiveness, and lack of proper focus. But there are some men's associations with the encouraging stated purpose of being a "spiritual organization of diverse men committed to promoting unity, to build a sense of community and to contribute to improve family relationships." There are groups called "GodMen" and others called "Promise Keepers" who believe that a Godly man is one of integrity, is serving, loving, and forgiving but also bold and as wise as Jesus. They seek to share intimate thoughts and feelings on practical daily life. The defining slogan of the Catholic Men's Fellowship is that "all growth occurs in relationships." The definition for "fellowship" is accepted as "men sharing their experience of God in their daily lives." Most often, though, the role and function of church men's associations or groups remains vague and uninspiring and consequently not well supported by the men in the congregation.

A men's fellowship group may provide men with the space they need and provide an entry point to the church for men who do not normally attend Sunday services. For men who do attend church, it may provide the opportunity to deepen the personal relationship with Christ through relationships with others as the gospel comes alive in the shared ordinary and difficult events faced on a day-to-day basis. It is an opportunity also for the development and nurturing of authentic Christian relationships in church, in the family, in the workplace, and in society at large.

Men have so much to offer, as protectors of society, as husbands and fathers, as grandparents, as role models. They have unique skills and interests and long for opportunities for these to be positively recognized. At the same time, men are under enormous pressures and expectations in the workplace and in the home. They frequently feel misunderstood, unappreciated, and blamed for all that is wrong—both the things within their capacity to respond to and those outside of their ability. The cultural norm of not showing feelings may leave them without support structures and mechanisms to cope with failures, upsets, and unrealistic expectations and to find the appropriate healing. Anger may be suppressed in the workplace only to erupt in the home, creating varying degrees of relationship damage. Men are at high risk of HIV infection when coping strategies are not in place; when the solution to marital problems is sought outside of the marriage; when there are peer pressures and the influence of alcohol.

Men also are socialized in ways that may increase their risk to HIV infection. It is common to find situations where men are raised to be macho, dominant in relationships, and ensuring the subordination of women. Male dignity comes with dominance and social power is accepted as the norm. This does not produce mutually enhancing relationships, and having multiple relationships is seen as a symbol of hegemonic power.[19]

Men seldom have health-seeking behaviour and are greater physical risk-takers, putting them more in the line of danger. Depression also is seen as a weakness and hence men frequently fail to deal proactively with early stages of illness. This again increases their vulnerability.

The church has a unique opportunity to offer this safe space, appropriate trainings, discussions, and support to help men feel heard, revitalized, and spiritually strengthened through the interactions of mutual support with other men, perhaps in similar circumstances.

Example: Catholic Men's Fellowship Groups of Greater Cincinnati

- It is men *ministering* to men in fellowship.
- It is a group of men who *pray* together, but it is not just a prayer group.
- It is a group of men of *faith*, but it is not just a faith group.
- It offers *social interaction*, but it is not just a social group.

- It studies the *Bible*, but it is not just a Bible study group.
- It offers *support*, but it is not just a support group.
- It discusses *various issues*, but it is not just a discussion group.
- It is aware of *religious issues*, but it is not just a religious action group.
- It considers *social issues*, but it is not just a social action group.

By creating a "safe space," where it is agreed that shared stories remain in confidence, and where no one is the expert, there is possibility for deeper engagement on issues that affect men in their day-to-day lives, positively and negatively, and the opportunity for growth in relationship with each other and with God. The group can decide on their vision and mission and recognize both the strengths and opportunities that exist amongst such a group.

Churches can explore principle issues of concern to men in their day-to- day lives, especially those that are likely to pose risks and render them vulnerable to HIV and ultimately to the impact of AIDS. Through a participatory process, men within their groups or clubs may be assisted to:

1. Describe what their vision or dream is for their lives, for a truly caring and supportive church, and for better communities for themselves and for their families, particularly as men in today's society and in an era of HIV and AIDS. What would it take to achieve this vision? What strengths are there amongst the individuals and church and amongst the social networks?

2. Identify the barriers to achieving this. What risks are there, including the risk of HIV infection? Identify principal issues of concern that pose risks to the men and ultimately may render them, or their families and those close to them, vulnerable to HIV and the impact of AIDS. For example:

a. *Priority issues/risks faced by men*:

- Cultural norms and expectations which are deeply ingrained in society. How to interrogate such cultural expectations as well as negative socialization, which leads to hurtful relationships.
- Financial pressures and expectations from so many sources and lack of skills in budgeting and financial management leading to stress, difficulties, and conflict.
- Pressures at work and at home, including extended family.
- The "father wound."
- Temptations!
- High stress leading to domestic violence and alcohol abuse.

- Extramarital "relief."
- Men's health issues—men frequently fail to look proactively after health.
- Gender paradigm beliefs that men should not do "women's work"; women should be subservient to men and not question men nor expect men to share information.
- Lack of skills in conflict resolution and anger management, leading to inappropriate or regrettable consequences at home, at work, and in society.
- Peer pressure and expectations.
- Lack of leadership skills.
- Lack of communication skills and skills in building/fostering relationships.
- Limited understanding of what love is and how it can be best expressed.
- Caring for HIV-infected relatives.
- Unfaithful wives.
- Discordant couples and issues of continued sexual relationships with each other, as well as problems associated with having children under these circumstances.
- Dealing with stigma associated with HIV.
- Dealing with grief and loss.
- Alternative sexual orientation with associated stigma.

b. *Knowledge of the men about risks and where to find information and/or help.* Do not assume that men have all the answers and information on risks, or that they already know where to find such information or help. Explore this area with them. Build on strengths that are already there.

c. *Current coping mechanisms and skills of the men to deal with the risks.* Ability to:
- Identify issues and thus risks
- Reduce risks and address issues at stake
- Prevent issues (e.g., seek appropriate training, support structures)
- Mitigate against impact
- Receive support if affected

3. Dialogue on what they would like to do to improve the situation, to limit risks to HIV infection, and to reduce vulnerabilities.

4. Agree on what *can* be done.
- Prioritize the risks based on risk assessment and identified needs. Identify *at least three* and agree to work on them within the men's club.
- Map the services available: support groups, training options, and the like.
- Identify skills and resource materials needed by men to deal with identified risks.
- Design or redesign programmes to allow for frank and open discussions and sharing; visit with other men's groups; undertake Bible studies that focus on the agreed topic or issue; invite people living with HIV to share their experiences;

have knowledgeable people lead discussions in areas of difficulty; show films that address the risks, vulnerabilities, and ways of mitigating impact.

- Delve deep into the Bible; it is full of relationship stories and lived experiences of people demonstrating virtually every possible event likely to be encountered by most men. Promote the methodology of Contextual Bible Studies as a way of men understanding women's issues better as well as their own issues.

- Allow sharing of the lived experience of individuals, especially where a living faith is strengthening the person's ability to work through the ordinary and extraordinary events of life. A crisis may be a gift and a weakness may in fact be a strength. Seek solutions that do not increase risk but, rather, minimize it.

- Find strategic partners to accompany or strengthen the initiative where necessary.

5. Implement the agreed activities together.

6. Measure and document progress according to agreed benchmarks and share experiences.

Example: Men as "Protectors of Society"

Ambohimarina Faharetana Dorkasy/AFF (FJKM), about 20 kilometres from Antananarivo in Madagascar, has a support group, called a "Listening Group," where many women from the church regularly meet to be in solidarity one with the other and to hear each other's problems. In a country lacking counselling services, especially in rural areas, such a support group represents a lifeline to the members. They have raised a question and a challenge to the church:

If a woman reports abuse, the offending partner is sent to a tribunal and imprisoned. This creates serious economic and social problems for the abused woman, who is then loaded with guilt, so most women suffer on in the abusive relationship. Most of the men do not come to church so the church has little opportunity to challenge them. Few come as couples to the church for support; the women are usually on their own with their problem. Sometimes the partners beg forgiveness and promise never to hit their wives again but once they are drunk or angry, they again beat their women. What can the women do to protect themselves and to survive in this situation?

There is great need to engage the men who *do* come to church, to reach out to such men—in the workplace, in the community, in the places of recreation, in the bars—to help them understand that violence in any form is unacceptable and will not be tolerated. Churches could open their doors as places of safety for women and children in crisis times and to stand with them through the challenges they face. Men in the church can be role models and reach out to other men, for whom violence is seen as a right and a regular solution to their own problems, to show and share that there are other solutions. Caring and supportive groups of men can ensure that such women are taken seriously when they report their story and are not further humiliated (or further abused).

> Together, we walk into a police station and make sure their cases are taken seriously. I find satisfaction as they face their perpetrators in court and convict them. I keep on doing this work, because no child, no woman, no man, should have to go through the difficult process of seeking justice—alone. —*Njuguna Thuka*[20]

> Our experience has been that men with the right information on equality between men and women stand a good chance of helping other men to change. If you allow men to vent out their fears about gender equality, you can help them understand the issues. Men can use men-only forums, meetings and one-on-one interaction to talk to others about violence against women in order to influence change. —*Kennedy Odhiambo Otina*[21]

Examples: The Car Service Project

In a church in Illinois, USA, the men's group offers a car-repair service for single women and the disadvantaged who cannot afford regular service charges. By tapping into the skills of men, who are doing something they enjoy, they render a valuable service to those who would otherwise have difficulty in affording such assistance, and they have their own social support group in the process.

Pietermaritzburg Agency for Christian Social Awareness (PACSA): "uMphithi Men's Networks and Amadondana Men's Networks (Men's Guild)"

PACSA is an independent, faith-based, nongovernmental organization that has worked to achieve social and economic justice for over 30 years. uMphithi Men's

Network and Amadondana Men's Networks (Men's Guild), programmes of PACSA, focus principally on men in the church, empowering them to reach out to men in the communities.

Vision: A society free of gender-based violence where men's positive attitudes contribute in promoting gender equality, healthy lifestyles, and good relationships amongst men, women, and children. A society where men fear God and strive to please God every day.

Area of operation: PACSA operates in 35 churches in the Pietermaritzburg area of South Africa. Pastors are involved and commit themselves and their churches to the programme. A pastors' breakfast is held quarterly to report and assess the participation of the churches. Church men's and women's ministries are specifically invited to work with these programmes. These same groups also become members of the networks; for men it is the Amododana Network. Where there are no such ministries in the church, there are "men's champions" who represent their churches in the network. If there are broader community forums, members of the community are also invited.

Objectives:

- Opening safe spaces for men and women to dialogue and share on issues that affect each of them.
- Creating good relationships and dialogues on gender and HIV-related issues, which can actively transfer gender and HIV awareness into their communities on a regular basis.
- Encouraging healthy lifestyles.
- Men's spirituality programme: "It's about reclaiming the spiritual initiation of men through experiential journeying into true self, and creating wisdom and tradition for future generations."

Strategies: The strategy for community mobilization with men involves three integrated approaches:

- Awareness raising through dialogues, campaigns, presentations during the church service to raise awareness about the programme and to invite participation, and workshops and specific trainings.
- Community accompaniment—walking alongside. Start where men are and "walk with them" little by little. This avoids confrontation and reduces drop-outs.
- Help to build linkages between the members and with other organizations involved in working with men.

These three approaches combine a community-driven and community-rooted approach with building linkages, which should lead to the ultimate goal of building a movement for social transformation.

Method of community dialogue: Start with participants discussing an issue in a nonjudgmental space, and minimize the role of a speaker. Let them talk for themselves on the issues that most confront them.

Types of topics discussed: Gender dynamics and gender as it relates to culture and religion; men and their relationship with their own health; alcohol abuse and HIV issues; ways of improving relationships between men and women.

Advocacy: The following issues have been promoted:

- Safe medical male circumcision through ensuring improvement in the traditional "boys' initiation camps" in South Africa and proper counselling and preparation of the boys.
- HIV counselling and testing, promoting the voluntary dimension and follow-up afterward.
- "Not in Our Name"—Ukuthwala Campaign. This is a campaign involving men who reject any form of violence against women and refuse to be identified with those who perpetuate it as a norm, a right, as culture, or under any other form or excuse.

Outcome: The integrated approach has enabled community level leadership of men to be involved in gender work; linkages have built strong foundations with wide impact and credibility has been established so their voice in advocacy is heard.

If we do not transform our pain, we will surely transmit it.
—*Richard Rohr*

Example: Ecumenical HIV & AIDS Initiative in Africa (EHAIA): Engaging Men: Transformative Masculinity and the Church[22]

Since 2007, EHAIA workshops, research, and publications have confirmed the need to tackle sexual and gender-based violence (SGBV) as a major driving force of the HIV pandemic. This has led EHAIA to mobilize churches, theological institutions, and other faith-based sectors to intentionally "break the silence" surrounding SGBV with the same vigor and commitment as shown to the HIV pandemic. In particular, with the use of Contextual Bible Study (CBS) methodology the team has effectively demonstrated the extent of the problem not only in communities but also within families and in the church itself.

As EHAIA has intensified the use of Contextual Bible Study methodology in addressing the HIV pandemic and its linkage with sexual and gender-based violence, a new challenge emerged: the urgent need to scrutinize social and cultural gender norms and gender inequalities, sexualities, and homophobia. In the process, the focus on getting men on board and creating "safe spaces" where they could talk about themselves, their fears, their sexuality, health, and spirituality has become one of the cutting-edge issues within EHAIA. Initially, groups of men met to scrutinize processes of socialization and masculinities on their own but they quickly discovered the need to include women who, as mothers, sisters, aunties, and grandmothers, play critical roles in socializing children into whom they become. Hence the theme of "transformative masculinities and femininities" in theological discourse was born. The staff, together with participants, also recognized that Africa can no longer avoid addressing issues of sexuality in all its diversity.[23]

Participants at these workshops include religious leaders, defense force and prison chaplains, staff from correctional institutions, people living with disabilities, people living with HIV, organizations working specifically with men and fathers, academics, and others who acknowledge the need to address these issues. They are encouraged to examine gender and cultural social constructs and the consequences of these. They are also encouraged to challenge patriarchal ideology, which promotes and encourages the notions of power, domination, and control over the female sex, and to adopt positive, more life-giving masculinities and life-fulfilling relationships that promote the principle of gender equality and equity.

Religious leaders play an important role in promoting transformative masculinities. The Bible has been abused to justify power-dominated relations and the oppression of women. "Some perpetrators of sexual and gender-based violence maintain that religion has accorded them the right to do as they please with women."[24]

These workshops and consultations have been described by participants as "eye-openers," "liberating," and "challenging but inspiring," and the impact has seen a trickle-down effect through the various churches and organizations that the participants represent across Africa. Results include:

- The formation of many men's forums to promote a positive and healthy masculinity and to raise awareness and counter SGBV in all its forms.
- Transformative masculinity being included in rehabilitation programmes in prisons.
- School programmes initiated to sensitize young people on healthier gender roles and respect for the other, as well as zero tolerance for any form of gender-based violence.
- Activism against gender-based violence and accompaniment of those affected.

- Men becoming peer leaders in their places of work and recreation.
- Youth taking on the challenge of "say no to violence in any form."
- Strengthened personal, church, and family relationships.

8.7 Engaged Couples and Married Couples

In the era of HIV and AIDS, the "mantra" that seems to have been perpetuated by churches is "Abstinence before marriage and faithfulness in marriage" as the solution to avoiding infection with HIV. Unfortunately, as statistics are showing, abstinence before marriage and faithfulness in marriage is little protection unless it applies to and is honored by both parties and both parties undergo testing before marriage. It also does not take into account the other methods through which HIV is so readily transmitted.

What is of equal concern is that, while churches preach the good message of abstinence and faithfulness, too often little is done beyond the preaching to help people to abstain before marriage and to strengthen the marriage relationship so that the parties want to be and are enabled to remain faithful in their marriage.

Engagement

In an era of HIV, all couples seeking marriage should be encouraged to go together for counseling and testing, and to share their results with each other. It may be difficult for either party to suggest they go for HIV testing without causing suspicions or raising contentious accusations. However, someone outside of their relationship recommending they undergo an HIV test can bring a sense of relief to many who recognize the need but are afraid to broach the subject.

It should not be expected of the couple to share their status with the pastor but it is essential that they share their results with each other. Also, the pastor should not refuse to marry an HIV-positive couple or a discordant couple; it is their choice, but they do need to be supported and to be assisted to find the information they need to help them cope with the additional stresses and responsibilities such a union will present, especially with regard to prevention of HIV transmission, and the necessity to consistently use condoms in their sexual relationship.

Preparation for Marriage

A wedding is a day, a marriage is a lifetime. —*Anonymous*

Couples need to prepare personally and as a couple for marriage. Each will be entering this union possibly coming from different situations and backgrounds and will have different experiences, fears, values, and expectations. Good marriages do not just happen; they need to be developed.

"Engagement Encounter" is recommended for couples who are seriously considering engagement or are already engaged or recently married.[25] It involves a weekend of reflection and mutual (not group) discussion, whereby couples are shown communication and decision-making techniques they can use throughout their lifetime together, in a nonthreatening and meaningful way. It represents an opportunity to talk honestly and intensively about their future together, to explore and share their own attitudes and expectations and to discover a deeper appreciation of their relationship and God's call to unite in a permanent union, the sacrament of matrimony.

Among the possible subjects they should have an opportunity to discuss with each other are: ambitions, goals, and attitudes about God, sex, money, children, family, and their role in the church and in the community. By developing a positive relationship with the couples before their marriage, the pastor has the unique opportunity to walk with them once they are married and to help strengthen that relationship.

Marriage

> A successful marriage requires one falling in love many times,
> always with the same person. —*Mignon McLaughlin*

"Be faithful in marriage." This is a commonly bandied-about statement but seldom are couples given the guidance they need on *how* to remain faithful in their marriage. Approximately one-half of all married men and 40 percent of married women have at least one affair during their marriage. Why? Why do couples seek solutions to their problems outside their marriages and not from each other? How do they make their marriages better, rekindle their romance when it flags, and strengthen the bond of their marriage?

The excitement and novelty of marriage in time becomes replaced with the mundane, the ordinary, and increasing responsibilities and time commitments as children enter the equation. It may seem that there is less and less time for each other and balancing work with home adds to fatigue and frustrations. Additional financial pressures, mutual and sometimes unrealistic expectations, extended family demands, and poverty of communication between the couple adds to marital strain. Conflicts may be unresolved, disagreements may turn into arguments, and the suppressed tensions and harboured resentment may surface. What may have started out as a simple disagreement becomes cluttered with recall of past failures, past disagreements, family issues, financial problems, and so many other unresolved, stored-up tensions, and the language may turn to angry superlatives, expressed as "you *always* . . ." and "you *never* . . ." Nobody *always* does something or *never* does something, but in the heat of the moment, things may be said which are difficult to retract and damage may be caused which is difficult to resolve. A rift develops which may turn into a gulf if it is not bridged and some common ground is found where better understanding and communications come to the fore.

The adage that "The family who prays together, stays together" has a lot of wisdom, because in prayer there is confession and the seeking of God's healing touch to relationships and a realization of a mutual need before God. The other adage of "Never let the sun go down on your wrath" equally holds much wisdom.

Couples very often lack communication skills, especially when hurting or angry. It takes a conscious effort to keep the disagreement focused on the issue at hand and not drag in past failures and problems. It also takes courage to hear what the other has to say without becoming immediately defensive and it takes true love and gentleness to share disappointments without crushing the other and "scoring a point" in the process. It is hard to say "I'm sorry" and it is difficult to be the first one to say it. Love is a feeling, a longing, a desire, but most of all, it is a choice and sometimes it is hard to chose to love the other, who can cause so much hurt through harsh words, emotional neglect, or error. Love is also a commitment which may need assistance from the church to fulfill, through support, guidance, and appropriate accompaniment.

Moreover, "Men and women alike want the security, safety, and comfort of a committed love relationship, but they long for the passion that seems to come only from a new relationship or from an affair. They want the best of both worlds. What they are searching for is what may seem a contradiction in terms: hot monogamy."[26] How do they find what they are looking for within their marriage and not seek it outside of marriage? In the vast majority of relationships, the sexual intensity begins to fade after a relatively short time. It needs to be replaced by a more sophisticated, consciously created, but even more fulfilling form of passion and intimacy. "Studies show that married couples have the best sex. Why? Because God's design works best when there is complete intimacy—emotional, spiritual AND physical."[27] Yet couples often lack relationship skills and are ignorant about their sexuality. There is an inability to talk openly and often limited intimacy skills. Where do they get advice or attend seminars focusing on such aspects as improving communication skills, managing conflict, enhancing personal growth, family wellness, and mutual fulfillment?

Churches offering the sacrament of marriage need also to be able to provide ongoing emotional and spiritual support to couples. If the pastor is unable to provide such direction and support, he/she should know where to refer the couples.

"Marriage Encounter" or "Marriage Enrichment" weekends are highly recommended, whereby couples have opportunity, in a nonthreatening and confidential environment, to listen to presenters talking and sharing on different potential problem areas and sharing skills that may enhance communication and resolution of issues of conflict. After each session on a different topic, the couples are given opportunity to spend private time together, to discuss what they have learned, to share how it resonates with their own experiences, and to talk to each other, either through word or through written letters and subsequent discussion. This opportunity of giving each other undivided time and attention, hearing each other out without interruption and in a nonthreatening and nonexposing environment, has proved to be very liberating for couples who really do wish to strengthen their marriages and to "be on the same page" in the relationship journey. The exposure to skills that work in resolving conflicts, in communicating, in expressing appreciation, in giving and taking, in handling demands of in-laws and children, and so on, are empowering and life giving in committed relationships.

Several churches offer these retreats on a nondenominational basis. They are highly effective in strengthening marriages and in providing couples with effective communication skills to appreciate each other and to affirm their relationship, to deal with the demands of extended family and children, and to be able to express needs in a noncombative or defensive manner. In the process, they also find healing.

> Let all bitterness, and wrath, and anger, and clamour, and evil
> speaking, be put away from you, with all malice. And be ye kind
> one to another, tenderhearted, forgiving one another, even as God
> for Christ's sake hath forgiven you. —*Ephesians 4:31-32*

> A happy marriage is the union of two good forgivers.
> —*Ruth Bell Graham*

8.8 Parent Groups

Becoming a parent adds a completely new dimension to an individual and a couple's life. In most circumstances within the church, it represents the fulfillment of shared love and commitment and is a sharing in the divine creation of another human being. "Sons are a heritage from the Lord, children a reward from Him," says Psalms 127:3. In many cultures, while we look to eternal life in the hereafter, children represent the perpetuation of life in the here and now. Marriages without children are considered unfulfilled and may result in the divorce of the woman (as she is most often considered the cause of the infertility).

For this reason, women may risk everything in order to have a child, even their own health. When antiretroviral therapy was unavailable, an HIV-positive woman was advised not to have children, as pregnancy could further compromise her health status and there was a risk of at least 33 percent of having an HIV-positive child. Most often, particularly in Africa, this advice was ignored, even if it meant repeatedly giving birth to an infected child and subsequent traumatic loss of the child, usually in infancy.

Now, with the availability of therapy, known as Prevention of Mother-to-Child Transmission therapy (PMTCT) and now referred to as Elimination of Mother-to-Child Transmission (eMTCT), an HIV-positive mother who accesses appropriate and timely medication can have a significantly reduced risk of delivering an HIV-infected child (down to 2 percent). This has created new hope for many couples who long for a child, but are conscious of the huge responsibility and challenge of passing on the virus to the unborn child.

However, significant numbers of children are born with HIV and survive infancy who are now in adolescence or teenage years. These young people are facing additional problems, compared to the average uninfected youth, of coping with the responsibility and challenge of their HIV-positive status. It may mean coping with recurrent bouts of ill health, the discipline of regular lifelong medication which may or may not have additional side effects, confidentiality issues, stigma, discrimination and rejection on the basis of serostatus, and the added difficulty of emerging sexual desires and the requisite needs and responsibilities in terms of disclosure and decisions. They do not want to be "different" from their peers and the need to be accepted is very strong. Many parents of such children and young people do not know how to tell their children either of their own positive status or that of the child. They struggle with issues such as when, how, and what to disclose?

Discussing sex and sexuality with young people is a difficult subject for most people and it is even more difficult when there is the added dimension of HIV responsibility. Parents may require help in this area. If the church does not offer such assistance, it is important that church leadership encourages such parents to seek help and it would be very valuable if the leadership is knowledgeable as to where such help may be sourced.

Parents today often feel extremely challenged and lacking in parenting skills, especially with adolescents, teenagers, and youth. Young people are struggling to establish their identity in a fast-changing world. Rebellion against the established norms and value systems is common as youth often feel it is "out of touch" with their reality. They also often feel "not understood" by those in authority over them. Parents frequently feel at a loss as their values are rejected together with their advice and guidance. Yet numerous studies have shown that youth still rate highly the importance of their parents, especially the importance of their parents staying together. It has been shown, in fact, that youth rate this far higher than parents realize. In handling circumstances with difficult youth, it is really important that youth still feel personally valued and that, although they may at this time reject parental values, they themselves are still valued by their parents.

An unhappy child can become an unhappy adolescent and an unhappy teenager. Such a situation does not resolve itself without understanding and a deliberate effort by both parties to improve communication skills. Initially, though, the weight of responsibility may lie with the parents. Without effort, the gulf may widen, with parents giving up on their teenagers. Without positive input from significant people in their lives, youth turn more and more to peers for affirmation, guidance, and acceptance. Lacking life experience, this scenario leaves them more vulnerable to some very negative influences from both individuals and society with dire consequences in an era of HIV.

"Absent fathers" is an increasingly common phenomenon for youth today. Men's roles in children's lives are diverse and go far beyond biological fatherhood. "It takes a man to be a Dad."[28] There is serious need to encourage responsibility of fathers toward their children, especially their sons. There is an equally important need for positive role models for such children who lack the experience of a father figure and it is an opportunity for parents to minister to each other.

The church can play a role in providing space for parents to share their experiences, both positive and negative, and to facilitate training in communication skills, skills necessary to cope with the emotional trauma of their children's rejection, to find ways to bridge the gap, to learn to offer unconditional love, and to "be there" for their children when they are in need.

A practical response is to run workshops with parents and the older community members on adolescent development and sexuality of young people in today's context. This can be an empowering process to assist parents and older people to communicate with the children on their development, especially noting that sex and sexuality are normal aspects of development, and it is far better to discuss this with the children than to ignore it.

It is also an opportunity to discuss other critical matters and topics such as finding ways to equalize gender power relations, building respect for the other and for themselves, as well as underscoring the rights and responsibilities they have for themselves and for the other. Another topical area of discussion is on homosexuality and alternative sexual orientation. Children may ask about it. They are sure to encounter such issues at school, college, and university. Parents should take care not to promote homophobia or judgment and be honest about their own feelings and knowledge or lack thereof in this area. Discussions on this or any similar topic related to sexuality will neither promote nor encourage children to be anything other than what they already are but it will empower them to deal with their own questions and to respond sensitively and appropriately with others with whom they have discussions/contact in this area.

> Your children are not your children.
> They are the sons and daughters of Life's longing for itself.
> They come through you but not from you,
> And though they are with you yet they belong not to you.
> You may give them your love but not your thoughts,
> For they have their own thoughts.
> You may house their bodies but not their souls,
> For their souls dwell in the house of tomorrow,
> which you cannot visit, not even in your dreams.
> You may strive to be like them,
> but seek not to make them like you.
> For life goes not backward nor tarries with yesterday.
> You are the bows from which your children
> as living arrows are sent forth.
> The archer sees the mark upon the path of the infinite,
> and He bends you with His might
> that His arrows may go swift and far.
> Let your bending in the archer's hand be for gladness;
> For even as He loves the arrow that flies,
> so He loves also the bow that is stable.
> —*Khalil Gibran, "On Children"*

8.9 People with Disabililties

About 650 million people in the world (10 percent of the world's population) live with disabilities, and frequently encounter a myriad of physical, economical, and social obstacles. They often lack the opportunities of the mainstream population and are usually among the most marginalized in society. Often, women with disabilities are invisible both among those promoting the rights of persons with disabilities and those promoting gender equality and the advancement of women.[29] People living with disabilities are also the world's largest minority group that is also frequently the most neglected and the most stigmatized. Few people realize we *all* are vulnerable to becoming disabled ourselves, as a consequence of accidents or as a side effect of certain diseases or medications or aging processes.

An emerging issue is the relationship between HIV, AIDS, and disability: HIV itself has the potential to actually cause disabilities, temporarily or permanently, and certain medications used in the treatment of HIV may actually precipitate disability.

Disabled persons are at higher risk of exposure to HIV. Gender plays a significant role as girls and women with disabilities are especially vulnerable to sexual assault or abuse. Similarly, those with intellectual impairment and those in specialized institutions are also at particular high risk as they are unable to defend themselves or perhaps identify the perpetrator.

Existing HIV programmes on awareness, prevention, treatment, care, and support generally fail to meet their specific needs, often because of a false assumption that such people are not sexually active and do not engage in any risk behaviours associated with HIV transmission, including drug misuse. People with disabilities are no different from the general population when it comes to the desire for intimacy, for having a partner, and for raising a family. Men who are disabled face stigmatization at the level of their masculinity, both as self-stigma and from the community at large.

School enrollment for children with disabilities is particularly low and the subsequent low literacy levels, as well as a distinct lack in appropriate resource materials, make it even more difficult for them over time to access the information, knowledge, and skills needed to protect themselves from infection.

Services offered at clinics, hospitals, and in other locations may be physically inaccessible, lack sign language facilities, or fail to provide information in alternative formats such as Braille, audio, or plain language.

There is far less information available in vernacular or in a user-friendly format for people with special needs. For example: a deaf person has difficulty getting frank answers to personal questions without a complete loss of confidentiality as very few doctors are able to communicate directly with the patient through sign language.

Though blind people may be able to read Braille, there is scant information on HIV in Braille and even less is available that is written from a faith perspective.

A person with disabilities who is also HIV-positive suffers a double stigma and the barriers to accessing testing, counseling, treatment, and support are even greater. In places where there is limited access to medication, persons with disabilities may be considered a low priority for treatment.[30]

Rejection at multiple levels is common and the church may be complicit in this when we overlook their plight or do not specifically reach out to people with disabilities. They are often "invisible" in our societies, especially in our churches, where accessibility may be a problem for them, or we fail to cater for their specific needs. Even in most national programmes, if people with disabilities are not featured in the national strategic plans or policies, they do not appear in the budgets. Such persons are unlikely to come to us, but do we go to them?

The World Council of Churches programme, the Ecumenical HIV and AIDS Initiative in Africa (EHAIA), makes a concerted effort to have persons living with disabilities included in all programmes and trainings. They are encouraged to speak for themselves and to raise awareness amongst religious leaders as to their strengths, not just their challenges. Most religious leaders and congregants do not mean to stigmatize or be insensitive to the special needs of colleagues; it is often just ignorance and a lack of opportunity to engage with them to enable better understanding and thus to respond more appropriately and practically.

Examples: Ecumenical Disability Advocates Network (EDAN)

As the author of the letter to the Ephesians stressed: Christ came to tear down the walls (Eph 2:14). Whenever we consider the ways in which to respond to issues of disability, we do well to remember the walls that we have set up. All of these walls are so human, yet they contradict Christ's ministry of reconciliation; walls that shut people in or shut people out; walls that prevent people from meeting and talking to others.[31]

Ecumenical Disability Advocates Network (EDAN) was established in 1998 following the Eighth General Assembly of the World Council of Churches. It was adopted as a Programme of the World Council of Churches within the Justice, Peace and Creation team work in 1999 and endorsed to be an effective decentralized conduit for advancing the concerns of disabled people globally.

EDAN members believe that *all* people, with or without disabilities, are created in the image of God and called to an inclusive community in which they are empowered to use their gifts, irrespective of the physical state of their bodies and level of psychological functioning. Hence, their main purpose is to advocate for the inclusion, participation, and active involvement of persons with disabilities in the spiritual, social, and development life of church and society.

EDAN's goals are to maintain an active network of people with disabilities, to improve their situation by providing the space for their contributions and gifts to the ecumenical movement and the churches, and to hold up this network as a distinctive *ecumenical* contribution to new models of being the church.

A Letter from Nigeria

"Just *start* by doing something." —*Jessie Benobo*

"You asked what exactly I do in terms of my involvement with persons with disability. Sometimes I ask myself the same question and wonder if it makes any difference at all—it's all so small compared to the big picture especially without apparent sustainability structures.

"This is what I do right now—we have a unit in my local Presbyterian congregation called the 'The Specially Gifted Committee—The Supporting Hands.' Membership is open to all persons. The committee works with persons who are differently abled toward an inclusive worship in the church. There are three categories of disabilities in my church right now—the blind, the deaf and mute, and those with various kinds of physical challenges—some in wheelchairs. The committee arranges for pick-ups to and from church for those who need such, arranges for guides for those who are sight-impaired, and signers for the deaf and mute. Right now, many of them have officially joined the church in full membership and bring their gifts to the worship activities of the church. The main organist, John, has a physical disability, so does Nne in the choir. Franklin, who is blind, is on the teaching and preaching schedule of the church and officiates regularly in church. We have been able to advocate disability-friendly church structures so our new church building now has ramps for those in wheelchairs and space created for the hearing-impaired who need to sit together for signing during the church services and other activities.

"Special church programmes are arranged for them where they get to invite their families and friends to share worship with them and we have the deaf sing and dance to songs of praise. At the last programme tagged 'Night out with the differently-abled,' a visitor who is himself physically challenged was enthralled by the song-signing of the deaf and exclaimed that he had never seen the deaf sing and dance before. We also give opportunities for them to share testimonies in regular services. Five of us from the church are now learning the American Sign Language.

"Some of our adult members are not economically active—the society and government have no employability plan for persons with disability. Although the law states that companies, as part of their social-responsibility acts, should employ members with disability, this is not happening. Our efforts to seek avenues for self-employment or placements have been largely unsuccessful but we keep trying. On Sunday, the church provides special lunch for them—this provides a further time for bonding among them and discussing issues peculiar to them. Beyond the lunch, it gives time to talk and enjoy good company. We give the backing of a church family—a safe place they can call home and friends they can always count on. This support system is crucial for a society where families with persons with disability are often confused and isolated.

"The steps we are taking are still baby steps—slow and shaky—but they are steps and we are not stopping. We have succeeded in creating positive awareness that in my local church, members no longer stare embarrassingly at persons with disabilities; they are embraced and welcomed and share conversations.

"No courses relating to studies on disabilities or the church's responses to issues of care are offered in the theological colleges here. This is another area for advocacy for us here."

8.10 Other Groups in the Church

Those on the margins of our society are also on the margins of justice. —*Anonymous*

Tolerance gives space but does not embrace the needy, the stranger, the deviant, the pervert, or anybody whose style of life and values are not one's own. But love does—God's love goes far beyond mere tolerance. . . . While tolerance might overlook differences and disagreement, love goes beyond all that to see the person as a child of our Heavenly Father. Much of the church in some parts of the world is so divided on matters of what we should and should not tolerate—of who is acceptable and who isn't—who should be allowed in and who kept out. If only we could be more open and accepting, more tolerant of others. . . . NO!—if only we who follow Jesus could move beyond such tolerance and learn to love in the ways he showed us to. —*Ronald Nikkel*[32]

Within every society there are marginalized people—outcasts and rejects because of a different ethnicity, religion, culture, tradition, behaviour pattern, sexual orientation, disability, or previous offense. The church runs the risk of mainstreaming itself so much that it contributes to the marginalization of so many. We may "shoot the wounded" from our moral high ground and contribute substantially to stigma and exclusion, pushing people further into the margins of society.

Scripture is full of accounts of God seeing beyond the obvious and *never giving up* on people, whatever their deeds or circumstances. God is first and foremost a God of love as well as a God of justice and mercy. God expects nothing less from us. How will those perceived to be "different from ourselves" ever hear the good news or experience the love of God through God's people if we condemn and exclude? We run the risk of expressing judgment, often based on ignorance and preconceived rigid values that may not necessarily, in any way, reflect "the will of God."

There may be difficult issues to understand, in the light of our interpretation of Scripture, but it does not mean that we should not enter dialogue to try to understand and it does not mean that we should not also offer unconditional love—as we are called to do. We need to read compassion *into* the texts rather than *out of* the texts.

> Many in the church and society are caught in traditional cultural and religious condemnations of people because of their sexual orientation. Homophobia, not homosexuality, is a choice. We don't choose whether we are straight or gay, but we can choose whether we are going to be open, caring, and compassionate, rather than prejudiced bullies or bigoted church people. Does being born again lead us to greater inclusiveness or narrow exclusiveness?[33]

If stigma and, sadly, religiously based shame and guilt, results in people being afraid to access services or to use treatment, then the goal of universal access will not be possible. Compassion should transcend religious legalism, as so powerfully demonstrated in some of the healing miracles of Jesus.

Thus, in mainstreaming HIV and AIDS into encounters with such groups here identified, a similar process to that discussed for the other departments/ groups in the church can be applied in the same way. Namely, in consultation with the target sector or group:

1. Ask the group to describe what is their vision or dream for the future, especially in relation to their circumstances and the place of the church within those circumstances. How could this vision be achieved? What opportunities are there for such a vision to become a reality? What strengths are already there that can be

drawn upon, both from amongst the group themselves and from the surrounding support networks of families, friends, the church, and others?

2. Where are we now? What is the current situation and what barriers are there to achieving this goal? What priority issues are individuals (and the group) facing? What might pose risks to HIV infection? What might increase vulnerability to HIV and the impact of AIDS? Identify the principle issues of concern which pose risks to the sector and ultimately may render them vulnerable to HIV and the impact of AIDS. These can be looked at in terms of:

- *Priority issues/risks faced by the sector*. For many, this may be the difficulties in accessing, receiving, or achieving basic rights that others take so much for granted. Through dialogue, and offering a safe space for such discussions, greater understanding may be achieved and more solidarity between members of the group.

- *Vulnerability of the target group, particularly to HIV infection and its impact*: People on the margins exist in every society, in every country, and are to be found in most communities, including our church communities. They may just be less visible or choose to be less visible because of fear of rejection and discrimination, as well as a sense of self-stigma that often accompanies such people. Because society marginalizes them and they are most frequently recipients of stigma and discrimination, they are and can become some of the most at-risk populations for HIV infection.

- *Knowledge of the target group to risks and where to find help*: Where group members are experiencing discrimination or overt stigma, the ability to access correct information may be a great challenge and a source of fear. Much of the information available presupposes the recipient not only can read, but can read English.

- *Resilience and skills of the target groups to deal with the risks*: We must never forget that all people have strengths and a resilience that has enabled them to cope thus far in life. We do not come with solutions to be imposed but a desire to strengthen and affirm what is good and to help where help is called for. They may have much to teach us as well. Where there is a demonstrable lack of skills, a collaborative strategy can be devised to address this situation.

3. Dialogue with the group on what they would like to do.

4. Discuss what *can* be done:

- Prioritize the risks and focus initially on addressing *three* of the most concerning risks, in an agreed and most appropriate or helpful way.

- Map the services available within the vicinity of the church and in the community served.

- Identify the skills and resource materials needed by leadership of the sector.
- Seek out relevant partners, allies, and colleagues to build capacity and to fill gaps in the church's ability to respond, as well as to complement or supplement responses, as appropriate.
- Refocus activities to address these identified issues in a collaborative, appropriate, and compassionate way.
5. Implement the agreed activities.
6. Measure progress, document, and share the process with others to affirm, motivate, and encourage others in their similar quest.

Example: Service for the Sex Workers in Madagascar

"I was on my way back to the airport in Antananarivo, heading home after engaging with many faith groups in Madagascar. My taxi driver was very chatty and interested in what churches on the island were doing in response to HIV. He shared new insights, from the perspective and knowledge of a taxi-driver. 'Do you see that embassy building over there?' he remarked, as we drove along. 'Next door is a church which holds special services on Saturday afternoons for the sex workers. This is a poor island and for some women on their own, sex work is their only means of survival for themselves and their children. But these women also want to go to church. The Sunday congregation does not like to see such women coming into their church, so the pastor holds a special service for them on Saturday afternoons. So many people come, with their children, too.'

"I reflected: When did we make our churches into mausoleums for saints and they ceased to be workshops for all sinners? When did we turn our churches into exclusive domains for the select, where our sensibilities and our comfort zones are not challenged? If Jesus were here in the living flesh, in which service would we find Him?"[34]

8.11 Support Groups

> Churches are called to reflect God's love to all people who suffer,
> who are marginalized, lonely, neglected, and at times feel hopeless.[35]

Support groups take many forms and provide members with varying types of help, usually nonprofessional and nonmaterial, peer-to-peer, for a particular shared, and usually burdensome, problem. The help may take the form of providing and evaluating relevant information, relating personal experiences, listening to and accepting others' experiences, providing sympathetic understanding, and establishing social networks. A support group may also work to inform the public or engage in advocacy.[36]

Self-help support groups are usually organized and run by volunteer members while professionally operated support groups tend to be facilitated by paid professionals who do not share the same problem of the group members, and are usually found in institution settings such as hospitals, drug rehabilitation, correctional facilities, and the like.

HIV support groups tend to include more than psychosocial support but also focus on rights and access to services and treatment. They help members realize that HIV is a chronic though manageable condition that need not be an impediment to living healthy and productive lives. It need not be a death sentence. The importance of such HIV support groups help members overcome stigma, particularly self-stigma, discrimination, and the fear of rejection by spouses, family, and friends. Disclosure, especially to family members, is very difficult and support groups, through the shared experience of others, can help members through the process. Members frequently look out for each other, accompany each other in times of need, and are in solidarity with each other. For those who are personally affected by HIV, such groups are sources of helpful and practical information on dealing with the implications and impacts of HIV (and AIDS) and provide a sense of not being alone.

Example: Support Group for Gays and Lesbians, Holy Trinity Catholic Church, Braamfontein, Johannesburg, South Africa

The political and economic problems in countries across the African continent, particularly in Zimbabwe, have resulted in large numbers of people seeking both refuge and a better life in South Africa. In an environment which is not altogether welcoming of such foreigners, they face huge challenges in securing accommodation, employment, and accessing medical care. They also suffer discrimination, xenophobic attacks, and the general loneliness of being far from family and friends. For many, the church provides a place of comfort and welcome. These large numbers of refugees and migrants represent a broad spectrum of society and thus, in their midst, are also people of alternative sexual orientation. They may have become migrants *because* of their sexual orientation, having experienced great rejection and stigma in their home place. Their sense of "aloneness" can be even more acute, increasing their vulnerability, self-stigma, and distress. Some of them are forced by family and community members into a marriage; some are subjected to "corrective" rape by intolerant and aggressively hostile community members and frequently find little support from the police.

Amongst the churches who are reaching out to refugees and migrants there is a notable one in the city of Johannesburg: Holy Trinity Catholic Church, Braamfontein, which has shown considerable support and care for refugees. A few of these refugees, who are of an alternate sexual orientation, asked the parish priest if they might show a film[37] in order to raise awareness and to help congregants better understand the issues which they face. The film looks at the situation of homosexuality as experienced by parents of such children and of the young people themselves. It is an honest look at the many challenges and difficulties that gays and lesbians and their families face, and how Christians use and misuse Scripture in response to their sexual orientation. As the church was having an exhibition of the various activities undertaken by the church, it was agreed that they, too, could show their film. This opened up frank discussions; the necessity for a support group became evident and so it was started. At first the priest did not think there would be many takers, but before long the numbers of the group had grown considerably. Now they meet every fortnight and, in the safe space created by the church, they have been able to share their painful stories and to find that they are not alone. Members have supported each other in accessing medical services and in caring for those who are at a very low point in their lives. During the Lenten season, the priest invited the group to lead the Friday evening service on the Stations of the Cross. This is a spiritual privilege which meant a great deal to the members of the group, who experienced not only the love of the Lord as they served him but also the unconditional love and care of the priest and members of the congregation.

Lord, make me an instrument of Thy peace; where there is hatred let me sow love; where there is injury, pardon; where there is doubt, faith; where there is despair, hope; where there is darkness, light; and where there is sadness, joy.

O Divine Master, grant that I may not so much seek to be consoled as to console; to be understood as to understand; to be loved as to love; for it is in giving that we receive, it is in pardoning that we are pardoned, and it is in dying that we are born to eternal life.
—*Prayer of St. Francis of Assisi*

8.12 Specific HIV Activities

Most churches are involved in one or more specific area of response to HIV and AIDS. The problem is that many of these activities are not part of a definitive policy in the church and are frequently run by good-will volunteers from the congregation. Such programmes run the risk of collapse should these volunteers need to move from the church as the activities are largely dependent on their drive and presence. In mainstreaming HIV into the life and ministry of the church, these activities should be part of the official policy of the church, endorsed, and properly supported. The activities should be part of an overall strategy to make the church HIV-competent, to reduce risk to HIV infection, and to mitigate against impact. It is also empowering for the volunteers to know that their activities are endorsed and that the church is behind their efforts. Together with an official policy in the church, there should also be a specific budget line dedicated to such activities, to facilitate the process, to acquire the necessary skills and capacities, and to fund if necessary. The following represent some of the many programmes, specific to an HIV and AIDS response, which churches offer.

Meaningful Participation of People Living with HIV

> Do not judge and you will not be judged. Do not condemn, and
> you will not be condemned. Forgive, and you will be forgiven.
> Give, and it will be given to you. A good measure, pressed down,
> shaken together and running over, will be poured into your lap.
> For with the measure you use, it will be measured to you.
> —*Luke 6:37-38, NIV*

Pope John Paul II made frequent and emotional appeals to avoid discriminatory treatment of people living with HIV. In his visit to people living with HIV in a California hospital in the United States in September 1987, he held out the unconditional love of God himself as the guideline to be followed: "God loves you all, without distinction, without limit. . . . He loves those of you who are sick, those suffering from AIDS. He loves the friends and relatives of the sick and those who care for them. He loves all with an unconditional and everlasting love."[38]

Example: Retreats for HIV-Positive Persons and Carers of HIV-Positive Persons
In a rural area of Zimbabwe is a small Benedictine monastery, Christ the Word Monastery, serving the local population and being a beacon of light and hope to the vast surrounding area. For many years, the monks at this monastery have been offering retreats specifically for groups of HIV-positive people, or the carers of HIV-positive people, offering them opportunity to feel cared for, loved, supported, and refreshed. They do so in recognition of the many challenges faced, on a daily basis, by those who live with and walk with HIV and to affirm their dignity and values.

Frequently, when a person living with HIV shares his or her story, there is a tendency amongst the listeners to focus on the story with a critical evaluation of "How did he/she get it?" This is a judgmental way of "blame" or "shame" whereby the listener determines how much sympathy or empathy the speaker does or does not deserve. Instead of focusing on how this person is managing to live with HIV, with all the accompanying challenges, we may be viewing them judgmentally, based on our presumptive curiosity, instead of following Jesus' commandment to *love* and to love *unconditionally.*

"Nothing for us without us" is a statement often heard from HIV activists. It has great value. People living with HIV need to be involved in all stages of our planning process. We need to acknowledge their capacities and aspirations and not just their vulnerabilities and fears. They have the greatest experience of the virus and knowledge of its impact on the individual and family. They can frequently best identify what increases stigma and what brings solace. Hearing the shared experience of a person living with HIV can have a transforming effect on preconceived attitudes and prejudices and can be a motivating force for change. It brings the situation of HIV from the theoretical into the practical reality. Open and meaningful involvement of people living with HIV in programmes can also encourage others in similar situations, or who suspect that they might be, to break their silence and seek out testing, support, and care. It can thus, in itself, be part of a prevention strategy.[39]

At every level, from community to national to international, the benefits of a greater involvement of people living with HIV have been shown. Their participation in policy, programme design, and implementation has been instrumental in reorienting priorities, ensuring relevance and effectiveness, and increasing accountability. As advocates for intensified prevention efforts, people living with HIV have been successful in bringing a human face and voice to the epidemic, challenging complacency and denial, strengthening the call for urgency in the response, and moving governments and their leaders to action.

In association with the Global Network of People Living with HIV (GNP+), the African Network of Religious Leaders Infected or Personally Affected by AIDS (ANERELA+), and UNAIDS, the World Council of Churches developed a "Framework for Engagement," for greater participation of all living with HIV in the life of the church. This includes a series of three documents which give a comprehensive overview of the situation and guidelines on the way forward, based on positive experiences worldwide.[40] This document was followed up by a complementary document on "Partnerships between Churches and People Living with HIV/AIDS Organizations" to assist in fostering a mutually beneficial collaboration.

As ANERELA+ became more international in its engagement and membership, it was rebranded as INERELA+: the International Network of Religious Leaders, both lay and ordained men and women, who are personally living with or personally affected by HIV. Currently, there are over 3,500 members across five continents. INERELA+ works toward empowering its members to be open about their status or situation and to use their positions of respect within their faith communities to challenge stigma, break the silence around HIV, and provide delivery of evidenced-based prevention, care, and treatment services.

The World Council of Churches, the Ecumenical Advocacy Alliance, and many other faith-based agencies and churches have developed numerous resource materials to be used in congregations, to acknowledge the presence of those who are HIV-positive in their midst, to be inclusive and nonstigmatizing, and to build the capacity of all in the church to develop a greater understanding, to face the reality of HIV for all of us, and to embrace a more practical and appropriate response.

> We're not dying from the disease. We're dying from the stigma.
> —*Gladys, HIV-positive member, Reformed Church in Zambia*

> Stigma remains the single most important barrier to public action.
> It is a main reason why too many people are afraid to see a doctor
> to determine whether they have the disease, or to seek treatment
> if so. It helps make AIDS the silent killer, because people fear
> the social disgrace of speaking about it, or taking easily available
> precautions. Stigma is a chief reason why the AIDS epidemic
> continues to devastate societies around the world.
> —*Ban Ki-moon, Secretary General of the United Nations*

Example: From EMPACT Africa[41]

The following represent some of the key characteristics of a stigma-free faith community as identified by numerous churches and faith communities and currently being collated by EMPACT:

A Stigma-Free Faith Community . . .

1. Talks openly about HIV and AIDS, as well as related issues such as sexual behavior and gender inequality.
2. Consistently and repeatedly gives messages of compassion, not judgment, toward people living with HIV.
3. Describes HIV and AIDS as medical conditions, not punishment for immoral behavior.
4. Provides basic facts about HIV and AIDS, including methods of transmission, and treatment, and prevention.
5. Encourages all members to participate in the life of the faith community, regardless of HIV status.
6. Focuses on providing care and support to people living with HIV, rather than on how they became infected.
7. Encourages positive living through education and support groups for people living with HIV.
8. Actively encourages testing for all members and facilitates access to voluntary counselling and testing.
9. Affirms the individual responsibility of all members to know their HIV status and to refrain from behavior that risks transmission of HIV.
10. Works proactively with other organizations to address HIV issues in the wider community.

To the above, Canon Gideon Byamugisha[42] adds: "A stigma-free faith community is human rights sensitive and social justice focused to tackle not only unsafe behaviours and practices but also the unsafe socioeconomic, cultural, and infrastructural environments that make safe behaviours and practices difficult to adopt, unpopular, and rare, whilst making unsafe ones easy to adopt, popular, and almost routine."

Benchmarks on Meaningful Participation of
Those among Us Who Are HIV-Positive

1. How many of us are openly positive in our church?

2. How many of our leaders are openly positive?

3. Do we have a workplace policy that is conducive to those among us who are HIV-positive?

4. Is there one currently being developed or adopted?

5. Are those among us who are HIV-positive part of committees in our church?

6. Do those among us who are HIV-positive feel welcomed and embraced in the congregation?

7. Do we have retreats or capacity-building programmes for those among us who are HIV-positive?

Prevention

Prevention refers to activities which have been designed to protect individuals from HIV infection such as: increasing awareness, promoting safe behaviour to reduce vulnerability to HIV transmission, encouraging the use of key prevention technologies, promoting social norms that favour risk reduction, and addressing the key drivers of the epidemic.[43] Increasingly, the use of antiretroviral treatment therapy is also recognized as a prevention strategy.

While the church is involved in many different activities in response to HIV, prevention is the one area that has generally lagged behind. The church has tended to be more reactive in response than proactive. Many reasons have been suggested but perhaps it is because the principal routes of transmission—through sexual activity and through intravenous drug use with infected needles—represent areas that are not easily discussed in church without much controversy. Sex and sexuality are not topics one may hear from the pulpit, nor is drug use, unless in terms of condemnation. Issues of abuse and specifically sexual gender-based violence are even less talked about, yet these are key drivers of the epidemic.

For many years national governments and faith-based organizations have relied on the prevention acronym "ABC": *Abstinence* before marriage, *Be faithful* in marriage, and *Condomize* if necessary. A considerable number of churches focus only on the "AB" and will not even discuss the "C," equating it with immorality and sin. The ABC acronym, while it has had its place, implies that HIV is only transmitted sexually and can have very stigmatizing associations: "Abstain before marriage and if you can't, then get married and remain faithful. If you can't be faithful, then use a condom." One country went even further to add "D": "If you can't use a condom, then 'D'—Die!"

While acknowledging the value of "abstinence before marriage" and "faithfulness in marriage" as a solution to avoiding or containing the risk of HIV infection, there are definite flaws in this simplistic approach within the context of many people's lives. There are children born with HIV, as a consequence of an infected parent. The message of abstinence and faithfulness has no relevance in their lives as they are already infected. Abstinence is not a realistic option for the millions of women and girls who are in abusive relationships, or those who have been taught always to obey men. People who do not abstain should do everything possible to reduce risk, including using condoms. A considerable amount of effort needs to be put into empowerment of women and girls and in advocacy against sexual and gender-based violence.

Abstinence until marriage does not always ensure safety, because marriage in itself provides no protection from infection. Many people are unsure of the HIV status of their partners, and those who are faithful cannot be certain that their partner is maintaining the same commitment.

Marriage has become an unsafe place as many faithful women are infected within their marriage. Some 40 percent of new infections in South Africa take place within the marriage. In the absence of HIV testing, those who are faithful in marriage but who are already positive continue infecting their spouses, reinfecting themselves, and infecting their subsequent children also. If an HIV-positive person responsibly purchases condoms to ensure that the virus is not passed onto the spouse, it is most often assumed by observers that the condoms are being purchased for acts of immorality.

"Faithfulness" is only protective when neither partner is infected with HIV, or both are mutually aware of their serostatus and respond appropriately, and both are consistently faithful. UNAIDS alerts that the approach is "of limited value" to many women and girls, as they cannot negotiate safe sex with partners or choose to abstain from sex.[44]

The ABC acronym does not take into consideration other forms of HIV transmission such as infection through blood products; sharp, unsterilized instruments; mother-to-child transmission in utero, during delivery, or through infected breast milk; children born HIV-positive who have never engaged in any sexual practice yet are positive; and infection through rape. HIV-related stigma and discrimination are found in all societies and can lead to social isolation and loss of family support. Fear of such prejudice can result in people failing to be tested for HIV, or not returning for their test results and thus not accessing the life-saving services and continuing to transmit the virus to an unsuspecting partner.

In 2003, the African Network of Religious Leaders Living with HIV and AIDS coined a new prevention approach with the acronym "SAVE" intended to encompass a far wider range of prevention needs.[45] This was later adopted by Christian AID for its HIV-prevention programmes.[46] This acronym is now being widely promoted as it is more inclusive, less stigmatizing, and encompasses so much more in the prevention message: SAVE is comprehensive—"It encompasses all evidence-based HIV prevention methods." SAVE is an acronym that stands for:

S: Safer practices

- Abstinence before marriage; mutual awareness of serostatus and faithfulness in marriage; and condom usage where there is a discordant couple or both are HIV-positive to prevent infection of partner or reinfection by partner.
- PMTCT+: Prevention of mother-to-child transmission through HIV testing of the mother in pregnancy and treatment to protect the unborn baby against acquiring HIV from an infected mother. It also involves considerations about breast feeding during the first six months of the baby's life. PMTCT+ aims to ensure the mother is also provided with the necessary antiretroviral therapy to prolong her life. Fathers of the children should also be tested and treated as applicable.
- Safe blood products: tested and HIV-free blood transfusions.
- Safe protection from blood contamination: gloves, sterile equipment, razor blades, piercing/tattoo equipment; syringes and needles, injections.
- Safe needles: needle exchange programme.
- Safe injections.
- Safe medical male circumcision.[47]
- Safe microbicides and vaccines research.

A: Access to:

- Treatment for: opportunistic infections, tuberculosis, and sexually transmitted infections, pre- and post-exposure prophylaxis, prevention of mother-to-child transmission.
- Antiretroviral therapy: both adult and pediatric.
- Adequate and proper nutrition.
- Appropriate information, which includes education on: HIV and its effects, modes of transmission, key drivers of the epidemic, sexual reproductive health, sexuality, relationships and responsibility, behaviour change, understanding of the risks of multiple concurrent partners, testing and treatment, nutrition, etc.

V: Voluntary, routine, stigma-free HIV counselling and testing.

E: Empowerment:

- Of children, young people, women, men, families, communities, and nations living with or most vulnerable to, most at-risk, and most affected by HIV and AIDS-related infections.
- To understand and respond appropriately to the negative social, economic, cultural, educational, political, and religious factors that influence behaviors and practices and may expose people to HIV risk and vulnerability.

The SAVE message, in its inclusive approach which recognizes the three main routes of HIV transmission—unsafe sex, unsafe blood contact, and mother to child—gives more space for collaboration between varying sectors in the response to HIV prevention and for care and support. It also reduces stigma and discrimination against people living with HIV and enhances their meaningful involvement "in positive living, positive prevention and treatment initiatives (not as problems to be avoided but as partners to be appreciated, involved and empowered)."[48]

Benchmarks on Competence: Prevention

Addressing prevention of HIV in a holistic manner and making us less vulnerable:

1. Is human sexuality addressed in a sound, forthright, and scientific manner and addressed to different age groups?

2. Do we discuss the social factors that can make us vulnerable to HIV?

3. Do we deal with cultural practices within our own society that enhance our vulnerability or protect us?

4. Do we reach out to those among us who are vulnerable in our communities or do we behave as if such a population does not exist?

5. In our education and activities on prevention, do we complete our information with scientifically proved and evidence-based methods such as use of condoms, clean needles, and clean syringes?

Counselling and Testing

HIV counselling and testing (HTC) is a critical entry point to life-sustaining care for people with HIV, a key element prior to treatment and essential for prevention of vertical HIV transmission and HIV transmission to others. Since HIV-antibody testing first became available, the World Health Organization (WHO) has advocated for people, especially those who think they may be at risk for HIV, to voluntarily seek out HIV testing and counselling. The cornerstone of WHO's guidance on HIV testing has remained constant for 20 years: confidentiality, informed consent, and access to counselling. Programmes in many countries offering client-initiated testing and counselling (CITC)—often referred to as voluntary counselling and testing (VCT)—have successfully informed individuals about HIV and prevention measures, and offered HIV test results, counseling, and referral for ongoing care and support to millions of individuals.

In many high-prevalence countries, however, fewer than one in ten people with HIV are aware of their HIV status. Reaching individuals with HIV who do not know their serostatus is a global public health priority and, more and more, the recommendation for *universal, systematic* offers of HIV testing and counselling is seen as an important step to achieving the goal of universal access to care and treatment for all people with HIV. HIV testing also provides an important opportunity for HIV prevention becoming accepted.[49]

Today, globally, only 40 percent of people with HIV know their HIV status. Up to 50 percent of HIV-positive people in ongoing relationships have HIV-negative partners (i.e., they are in serodiscordant relationships). Of those HIV-positive individuals who know their status, many have not disclosed their HIV status to their partners, nor do they know their partners' HIV status. Consequently, a significant number of new infections occur within serodiscordant couples.[50]

Since the serostatus of one partner has potential life-threatening implications for the other, and to ensure both partners together understand and decide on mutually agreed courses of action, it is recommended that *couple* HIV testing and counselling (CHTC) is promoted. Together they test and mutually disclose their results in an environment where a counsellor or trained health worker is on hand to offer support and advice on a range of prevention, care, support, and treatment options.

Many churches provide counselling as an accompaniment to testing, both pre- and post-testing. Frequently also, churches makes their structures available for counselling and testing to be undertaken on site. Where governments appear to provide all the services in terms of testing and treating, many churches have found an opportunity to be critically involved by offering the counselling service and for clients to be referred to the church for support and ongoing accompaniment.

Premarital testing is highly recommended and the couple should be advised to mutually share their results, so that they can make informed decisions about their future. The pastor should not expect to be told the results and neither should he refuse to marry the couple if one or both are HIV-positive—it is their decision—however, it would be a mark of love and a sign of HIV competence if the pastor were to offer to accompany the couple, whatever their status and whatever their decision.

Churches can organize to have HIV testing and counselling done on site, whenever there are workshops or other events. Pastors can lead by example to "know your status" and other congregants may feel more comfortable testing with others in the local congregation as opposed to a public venue.

WCC-EHAIA offers HIV counselling and testing during all major workshops. Religious leaders are encouraged to "know their status" and to experience personally the testing and counselling process: again, lead by example. Many religious leaders have expressed gratitude at this opportunity as they feel uncomfortable to be seen testing in a public venue, as stigma still remains so high. They are afraid their reputation will be compromised and damaging presumptions may be made that will quickly circulate. In numerous questionnaires with religious leaders and congregants, conducted by EHAIA in workshops, participants regularly raise concerns about gossip in the church, and that the pastor's wife is frequently the source of much of the gossip, based on her knowledge of "confidential discussions with the pastor"!

Churches and faith-based organizations across Africa, such as Philippi Trust in Namibia, offer counselling training courses, either run by the church itself or through the expertise of trained personnel and often utilizing the premises of the church. Pastors frequently cite the need for such trainings because pastoral accompaniment of persons living with HIV or personally affected by HIV is multidimensional; since many express lack of appropriate skills to cope.

Examples: Lesotho Church Offering Its Venue as a Testing Site

An Apostolic Faith Mission Church in Maseru, Lesotho, sought ways that they could respond to an ever-growing epidemic of HIV. Lacking expertise within their own ranks they opened up the church to a nongovernmental organization that specifically focuses on counselling and testing, to operate from within the church premises on a regular weekly basis. The church announced it from the pulpit, encouraged parishioners to avail themselves of the service, and offered ongoing accompaniment of any or all who found that they were personally affected by the virus. Over a period of several months, growing numbers of people from the surrounding community came for testing, expressing comfort with testing "at church." In the process, the church became increasingly aware of the impact of AIDS in the lives of many congregants and people living in the surrounding community. An orphan outreach and support programme was then initiated, involving many volunteers from the church. Incrementally, these activities, carried out in a nondiscriminatory and nonstigmatizing environment, broke down many barriers between community members and members within the church, strengthening relationships, as faith was demonstrated in action.

"I thought I was the expert on counselling."
—Statement of a counsellor in Karnataka, India

"In 2011, I visited a hospital/hospice in North Karnataka state, India, where I engaged with staff, patients, and patient's families and caregivers alike. One of the staff members, a highly trained HIV and AIDS counsellor with many years of experience, recounted a personal experience which was deeply challenging. She said: 'One day two sisters in their twenties came into the hospital. The older one obviously had full-blown AIDS and she was accompanied by her younger, healthy sister. I knew I had some serious counselling to do: the ill sister needed to understand and come to terms with her condition and to prepare for what was to come. The younger one needed to understand what was happening and the implications of the disease. I knew I had my experienced work cut out for me. However, the older girl just kept crying for her [deceased] mother. Nothing I said seemed to make any impression on her. The younger sister, however, took the ill sister in her arms, cradling her and singing gently to her whilst she caressed her hair. It had a soothing effect on the ill woman and she seemed to find peace in those gentle gestures. All my training and knowledge was nothing against the wisdom of the younger sister, who showed love and was a mother to her dying sister. It made me realize that we sometimes see ourselves as such experts in dealing with HIV and AIDS that we overlook the power of touch, the beauty of silence and empathy, and the healing power of love that transcends the multiplicity of our words.'"[51]

Benchmarks on Competence: Counselling and Testing
Opportunities within our communities' own sacred space to test for HIV in a supported, confidential, and secure manner:

1. Do our leaders and members know where testing is being done?
2. Is the congregation connected to and able to refer members to testing facilities?
3. Do we have facilities within our own structures for testing?
4. Do we maintain confidentiality?
5. Can discordant couples (i.e., when one partner is HIV-positive and the other is negative) who are among us get sound advice and support from our congregation?

Treatment

> Faith based organisations are a vital part of civil society. Since they
> provide a substantial portion of care in developing countries, often
> reaching vulnerable populations living under adverse conditions,
> FBOs must be recognised as essential contributors towards univer-
> sal access efforts. —*Dr. Kevin de Cock*[52]

Treatment is now the cornerstone of the response to HIV and has succeeded in turning a death sentence from HIV and AIDS-related illnesses into a chronically manageable illness—for those who have access to the necessary therapies, regimes, and nutritional support. Even further, there is emerging promising evidence of using a regime of antiretroviral drugs to prevent transmission of HIV: treatment as prevention.[53] The gap between diagnosis of HIV and access to appropriate treatment therapies needs to be narrowed as this delay is compromising the health of the individual and increasing the chance of infection of others.

Church health institutions are the medical arm of the church. For example: the Zimbabwe Association of Church-Related Hospitals (ZACH) provides 45 percent of all hospital beds in Zimbabwe and 68 percent of all rural hospital beds. As such, most of these institutions across Africa are involved in various levels of care, counselling, testing, CD4 measurement, HIV diagnostic testing for infants, ARV treatment and distribution, and nutritional support. In addition to providing health care, patients frequently identify church-owned health institutions additionally as important sources of compassion and support, where they experience less stigma and discrimination than in government-run facilities.[54] Some of these facilities were among the very first, in many countries, to actually offer antiretroviral therapy, ahead of national governments.

Through outreach, people personally affected by HIV and volunteers become "buddies" to those who are in need of antiretroviral therapy, accompanying them in the process, encouraging, reminding, assisting in treatment collection if unwell, and generally being supportive friends in times of need. This results in better treatment adherence and ensures the well-being of the affected person, as they do not feel so alone with their condition.

Churches, too, have in many instances becomes treatment centers, especially where such facilities are deficient or simply nonexistent in the surrounding communities. In addition, religious leaders have been encouraged to promote "treatment literacy" whereby congregants and members of the community are helped to understand the principles of treatment and nutrition, the benefits of treatment, and the essential need for compliance and adherence. Patients also need to be aware that tuberculosis frequently accompanies HIV and thus screening for TB may be included in the investigation and monitoring process.

Until very recently, it was believed that having an HIV-positive diagnosis did not automatically mean that the person concerned needed to start antiretroviral therapy. With correct nutrition, health, and lifestyle management and timely treatment of any concomitant infections, it was believed the person concerned might remain well, without initiation of ARV therapy, for many years. They would also be able to maintain a satisfactory CD4 count considerably above 350, which has been the identified as the cut-off level of the ability of the immune system to cope with HIV infection, below which is the high risk of progression to full-blown AIDS. Current scientific evidence, however, is suggesting earlier treatment, initially at a higher CD4 count and now irrespective of CD4 count. The reality, though, in most developing countries, is that the sheer cost and logistics involved will mean that this is not likely to happen under current funding restraints and vast numbers of HIV-positive people will need to remain as healthy as possible while they await access to antiretroviral therapy. Once they do start on therapy, both the patient and those closest to them need to understand the treatment rationale and importance of compliance. Hence, those who have regular contact and compassionate care and concern for the well-being of HIV-affected persons are being encouraged to become treatment-literate and to share this knowledge with those who most need to understand it. Organizations such as the Ecumenical Pharmaceutical Network have produced manuals to assist religious leaders to address the issue of stigma and discrimination and to learn how to care for those infected and affected, supporting them both to seek treatment and to stay on treatment.[55]

Examples: The Eastern Cape Moravian Church and HIV Treatment

A Moravian church in the Eastern Cape, South Africa, has introduced a programme whereby those who are on antiretroviral therapy take their medication at the same time as they would normally read the selected Scripture readings for the day. It is a way to ensure that there is regular adherence to the taking of the medication but it also "spiritualizes" the treatment. Treatment becomes a shared spiritual experience between God and the patient.

Churches Become HIV Clinics in South Africa

South Africa is a country that has been severely affected by HIV and currently has over five million people living with HIV. Political obstruction and vacillation meant that persons living with HIV were unable to access the life-saving ARV therapy which was available in other countries. The South African Catholic Bishops Conference initiated a programme of preparedness, in anticipation of ARV rollout. This involved increased training of counsellors and establishment of more testing sites, treatment for opportunistic infections, and preparation for treatment distribution and adherence. "Buddy" systems were introduced along with a creative use of volunteers, church buildings, and compassionate motivation.

As soon as the government announced that treatment could be rolled out, the Catholic Church was ready. Funding from the U.S. President's Emergency Plan for AIDS Relief provided the necessary means to screen patients and distribute antiretroviral medications and follow-up. "Armed with just parish buildings and the compassion of parishioners, the Catholic Church transformed churches into HIV clinics in the hardest-hit regions of the country."[56] With Catholic Relief Services support, the church is now providing HIV care and treatment to over 60,000 people living with HIV, and some 20,000 are receiving ARV from 14 primary sites and related outreach services in remote areas, with most facilities being parish churches. The intention is for a strengthened partnership with government and a transfer of this "high-quality HIV care to the public sector for long-term sustainability."[57]

Prevention of Mother-to-Child Transmission (PMTCT)

There are more than 40 million people living with HIV infection globally, 24.7 million of whom live in sub-Saharan Africa. Increasingly, women are disproportionately affected by HIV: 60 percent of HIV-positive adults in Africa are female, and the vast majority are women of childbearing age. Young women aged 15 to 24 are four times more likely to be HIV-infected than men of similar age; these are the years during which many women become mothers and begin to raise families.[58] Children and families are strongly affected by issues that affect women. The vast majority of the more than two million children living with HIV were infected through mother-to-child transmission.[59] The specific vulnerabilities of women to acquiring HIV infection, coupled with inadequate access to family planning and HIV prevention and treatment services, have resulted in an unabated worldwide pediatric HIV pandemic.[60] Children living with HIV are at high risk for morbidity and mortality early in infection, with almost half dying by the age of two if their disease is not properly managed.[61] Those who survive face the potential loss of infected parents, along with intermittent ill health and overwhelming stigma. In short, the effect of HIV on families, with women as the linchpin, has been devastating.

Faith-based organizations (FBOs) have maintained long-standing involvement in the area of prevention of mother-to-child transmission. In many countries, the church-related hospitals and mission facilities were among the first to successfully roll out PMTC treatment, even in very resource-constrained settings and in the face of initial skepticism on the reliability of the clients to adhere to treatment. A recent study of the Catholic HIV/AIDS Network (CHAN) shows that almost three-fourths of respondent Catholic Church-related organizations reported provision of a range of PMTCT services, which include voluntary counseling and testing, ARV treatment and distribution, CD4 count testing, HIV diagnostic testing for infants, and nutritional support for women living with HIV, as well as ARV treatment and nutritional support for children found to be HIV-positive.

With the launch of the 2011 UN *Global Plan towards the Elimination of New HIV Infections among Children 2015 and Keeping Their Mothers Alive*, faith-based organizations have been identified as key stakeholders in efforts to implement the plan and to reach the ambitious global targets. The following are five steps, suggested by UNAIDS in 2012, that religious communities can take to stop new HIV infections in children and keep their mothers alive:[62]

1. Support women to avoid HIV infection. A mother who is free from HIV cannot pass on the virus to her children.

2. Provide information in local faith communities encouraging and supporting couples to go together for HIV testing.

3. Support access to antenatal care and HIV testing and counselling for pregnant women and provide linkages to related health facilities and care.

4. Strengthen programmes to prevent new HIV infections in children—in line with national policies and protocols—in religiously affiliated hospitals and medical centres, particularly in rural areas.

5. Ensure coordination with national health systems addressing HIV prevention and treatment to enable pregnant women living with HIV to access the best possible antiretroviral therapy—for their own health and for their baby's health.

Example: Faith-Based Organizations and Prevention
Elimination of Mother-to-Child Transmission

Faith-based organizations have long been involved in the area of prevention of mother-to-child transmission of HIV infection. People living with HIV are increasingly trained and involved in peer education and support, encouraging pregnant mothers to seek and access necessary testing and treatment, and accompanying them in the process. Mission hospitals, in particular, have very often initiated and run programmes that extend beyond HIV testing and diagnosis, CD4 lymphocyte measurements, and appropriate antiretroviral therapy, to addressing the many social, economic, and psychological needs of HIV-positive patients, their families, and the communities in which they live.

These programmes include guidance on growing nutritional gardens, food support, and other income-generating activities in addition to numerous age-appropriate support groups. In all activities, concerted attempts are made to involve both the father and the mother and to strengthen the family unit.

Benchmarks on Competence: Treatment

The congregation facilitating and sustaining the access to life-giving treatment:

1. Do we as a community take steps to promote treatment literacy—like giving information, conducting seminars/workshops, and training of congregation members?

2. Do we know where we can refer pregnant women and their spouses to be screened and to benefit from the prevention of parent-to-child transmission of HIV and would we advise them to utilize the service?

3. Are we involved in dispensing of medicines and facilitating buddy programmes (i.e., individuals who are trained and committed to accompany a person in need)?

4. Do we provide treatment of opportunistic infections and antiretroviral therapy?

Care

> Then the King will say to those on his right, "Come, you who
> are blessed by my Father: take your inheritance, the kingdom
> prepared for you since the creation of the world. For I was hungry
> and you gave me something to eat. I was thirsty and you gave
> me something to drink. I was a stranger and you invited me in.
> I needed clothes and you clothed me. I was sick and you looked
> after me. I was in prison and you came to visit me." . . . The King
> will reply, "I tell you the truth, whatever you did for one of the
> least of these brothers of mine, you did for me."
> —*Matthew 25:34–36, 40, NIV*

Home-Based Care

> Home-based caregivers' impact was often found to be life-saving
> and life-preserving in ways that have been little examined in the
> social-scientific and public health literatures. —*Robin Root*[63]

Home-based care is one of the principal services offered by churches in the era of HIV and AIDS. It is a natural extension of a time-honoured service that involves visitation of the sick. Indeed, the principle of home-based care for people living with HIV or AIDS was started by a mission hospital, Chikankata, in a rural province of Zambia in 1987. The effectiveness of such a service was quickly recognized and acknowledged and the idea spread all over the world.

Home-based care, operated by churches or faith groups, is usually characterized by an informal service delivery that is usually run by volunteers, in response to a Christian mandate to "visit the sick" and out of the kindness of their hearts and in empathy with the suffering of others. The type of service offered may supplement the care already provided by family members or other primary caregivers or it may be the only external care that the person receives. Such care ranges from visitation of the sick or affected person(s), offering psychosocial and spiritual support, to actually undertaking a number of activities that include physical and medical support with food supplements, administering basic remedies and treatments, and other forms of custodial care such as cooking, cleaning, assistance with feeding, washing and toilet care, and supportive outreach to the children of those homes.

Currently most home-based care programmes focus on the needs of adults living with HIV in the household. It is far better to broaden the approach to assess and meet the needs of the children within the household as well. The impact of HIV and AIDS can drive families into severe poverty. Children may be absent from school, have compromised nutrition, or be assuming adult roles in the care of younger siblings and taking over household responsibilities. Some children may be facing the prospect of orphanhood. Relationships with the children can be established, referral systems tapped into, which may mitigate some of these needs, and parents can be assisted to identify who they wish to be involved in the care of their children when they are no longer able to do so themselves.

Examples: The Chikankata Care Experience: Zambia

Weddy Silomba, human resources and training manager for Churches Health Association of Zambia, reports, "Communities have capacity to respond to HIV/AIDS in spite of the overwhelming number of HIV/AIDS infections at present. Externally supported programs are needed that seek to alleviate the suffering of the orphans, vulnerable children, and PLWHA [people living with HIV/AIDS]. However, what should not be ignored is the inherent capacity to care that exists in the neighborhood and communities. Care programs should seek to create a process of 'being present with' clients to bring about hope, healing and wholeness. This arises from a respect for and appreciation of the internal strengths and skills of communities to identify and address a variety of problems. As seen from the Chikankata situation, it is this active engagement in care manifested in oneness with communities that has motivated communities to embrace concepts of care and prevention with passion. The community counseling process allows for openness, flexibility and respect for comparative advantages. The structure of the care and prevention teams is a unique tool with which to foster care and prevention and development in the context of AIDS prevention."[64]

St Joseph's Care Centre:
Sizanani Village, Bronkhorstspruit, South Africa

Our mission is to serve people who are ill, at the least possible cost to themselves, in cooperation with their family, neighbours and community members. We aim to promote open non-judgmental attitudes towards people with HIV or AIDS. We value human life, both the unique individual and the community as a whole.

Through this service, people with a terminal illness, especially those with AIDS, are cared for in their homes. People who are caring, understanding, loving, discreet, and committed are chosen to be caregivers in the community. They are trained in basic nursing skills with emphasis on palliative care and counselling. They live close enough to the patients to visit them regularly. Caregivers are trained to maintain confidentiality, so that the patients and families feel comfortable, knowing their privacy is protected. A coordinator guides and supervises a number of caregivers in a specific area. When necessary, referrals are made to hospitals and clinics and hospices. Caregivers are guided by professional staff in their work and supported by a "Care for the Carers" programme. The services offered include:

- Home-based care outreach programmes for people with a terminal illness in their homes
- Nutritional and medical assistance
- Transport to clinics and hospitals, if this is not available to patients and their families
- A counselling service for those infected and affected by HIV
- Ongoing training related to HIV and AIDS nursing skills, project management, budgeting, and report writing
- A support programme for caregivers

The work is done in partnership with government departments, local authorities, clinics, hospitals, church organizations, and other NGOs.

Hospice Care

Hospice is not a place so much as a philosophical approach to the care of patients and their families who are dealing with end-of-life issues when a cure is not possible for the illness that is faced. It is a model of care that provides pain relief, pain control, and system management as well as emotional care and spiritual support for both the patient and the entire family. It is not giving up on life but, by taking control, it is choosing quality of life with dignity for the remainder of the patient's life. Palliative-care programs seek to bring such compassionate services to patients earlier in the course of the illness. Palliative care is also very appropriate within home-based care as it utilizes affordable medications and the family is empowered to care effectively for their own members in the familiar home setting.

Examples: Overstrand Care Centre[65]

The Rev. Pamela Parenzee at the Parish of St. Andrew's Hawston in the Cape, South Africa, initiated a hospice in the community linked to the church. It is a place for terminally ill people that provides a peaceful place to rest and, for others, a home in which to die with dignity. The hospice operates with a group of caregivers who look after the sick and work in the kitchens. The hospice also has a sustainable food garden where all nutritional vegetables for the meals are grown.

Mashambanzou Care Trust[66]

Mashambanzou Care Trust was founded in Zimbabwe in 1989 by a Catholic nun, Sr. Noreen Nolan, of the Little Company of Mary. Having worked in rural areas and having seen the impact of AIDS she initially started a terminal-care ward attached to a Catholic-run private hospital in Harare. The pressing need for such care in the high-density areas led to the founding of a centre on the outskirts of the city to cater to the large numbers in need of terminal care.

In those early days of no antiretroviral therapy, men and women and young people, suffering alone and terribly from the effects of often untreated AIDS-related illnesses, were taken into the hospice to receive treatment, care, and support. Once their condition improved sufficiently, they would return to their homes and be followed up by the home-care teams. Some would end their days in the centre, receiving loving care and support, which enabled them to die in peace and with dignity.

Over time, Mashambanzou trained over 250 volunteers in most of the high-density areas around Harare. The centre now offers a wide range of services including: a drop-in centre; a play centre for the children of patients, pre- and post-test counselling; a terminal-care centre that can accommodate 22 patients; home-based care and treatment accompaniment; and bereavement support and counselling. Referrals come via Harare clinics, hospitals, other care organizations, or word of mouth. Volunteers come mostly from the churches.

In one year alone, four home-based care teams, each with a sister and a counsellor, visited some 8,350 patients in their homes. In the same year, 1,506 orphans received assistance.

Prison Care

> "I was sick and you looked after me. I was in prison and you came
> to visit me." Then the righteous will answer Him, "When did we see
> you sick or in prison and go to visit you?" The King will reply, "I tell
> you the truth, whatever you did for one of the least of these brothers
> of mine, you did for me." —*Matthew 25:36b, 37a, 39, NIV*

> Jesus Christ, the prisoner, the embodiment of God's love for the
> down and out as much as for the up and out. . . . Jesus continues
> to embrace politicians and prisoners; rich and poor; liberals and
> conservatives; Buddhists, Hindus, Muslims, Jews, and Christians;
> unbelievers, believers, and atheists; straights and gays and in-
> betweeners; you and me and every human being with His irresist-
> ible and redemptive love. —*Ronald Nikkel*[67]

Every year some 30 million men and women spend time in prison. One-third of
the prison population is in pretrial detention and presumed to be innocent. Most
incarcerated people will return to their community, many within a few months to
a year. HIV prevalence in prison can be two to ten times—in some cases up to 50
times—higher than in the community. HIV and tuberculosis are the main causes
of death in most prisons. Antiretroviral, tuberculosis, and drug-dependence treatment are often interrupted when people are arrested, await conviction, and enter
the prison system or when they are released. HIV in prison settings affects all
regions of the world, especially sub-Saharan Africa, reflecting the high prevalence
in the general population, and in Eastern Europe and Asia, reflecting the high
prevalence of injecting drug use.[68]

People in prison are marginalized, stigmatized, and often rejected by society.
Where they are imprisoned far from home, they seldom receive family visits and
this increases their sense of isolation and rejection. The Christian community
worldwide is compassionately engaged in ministry to the poor, the disadvantaged,
and the marginalized, including those in prisons.

Men, women, and children in prison, those released from prison, and families
on the outside, are rightly included among the needy and must be included in the
ministry of the church. Through acts of compassion and selfless service, thousands
of Christian volunteers visit local prisons, support released prisoners, and provide
ministry to prisoners' families. The need is great. Jesus called it serving the "least of
these." Christians who voluntarily go into prisons, or work on the outside with ex-

offenders and prisoner's families, make up an army of carers demonstrating the love of Christ to the marginalized. The active involvement of the Christian community is vital for prison ministry. Such ministry would not exist in the form, breadth, and depth that it does without the engagement of the church.[69]

There are many resources to assist with engaging the church, from worldwide organizations such as Prison Fellowship International to chaplaincy programmes in prisons.

Example: Transformative Masculinities and the Lesotho Correctional Services
The World Council of Churches—Ecumenical HIV and AIDS Initiative in Africa (WCC-EHAIA) has, for a number of years, been engaged in forums for men (and women) on "Transformative Masculinities." In 2010, senior members of the correctional services in Maseru, Lesotho, were invited to attend and share experiences of working with large numbers of men who find themselves on the wrong side of the law. The forum proved to be transforming *for the staff* themselves, who often find they are living and working under a great deal of stress and, as a consequence, alcohol abuse and domestic violence is common. The same staff then instigated a similar training for the staff of all the correctional services in Lesotho, with very positive and transforming results. Transformative masculinity topics are now included in the rehabilitation programme for offenders. In addition, sensitization sessions have been undertaken with many churches, with high school students, and with staff of the police stations.

Benchmarks on Competence: Care
Caring for those of us in our congregation and in our community who are hurting with HIV:
1. Do we have home-based care programmes? *(none; or first-level care: occasional—visits once every two weeks, or less frequent visits, and material support; or second-level care: regular visits, more fortnightly visits, and material support; or comprehensive-care programme which includes care, prevention and treatment, and holistic support)*
   2. Do we provide nutritional aid?
   3. Do we provide legal aid to those among us who are HIV-positive or marginalized?
   4. Do we see prevention as part of care?

Sexual and Gender-Based Violence

Gender inequalities fuel and exacerbate HIV epidemics. Although gender issues vary across communities and countries, power imbalances, harmful social norms, violence, and marginalization affect both women and men across the world.[70] They increase people's vulnerability and limit their ability to prevent HIV infection.

Gender-based violence (GBV) is an umbrella term for any harm that is perpetrated against a person's will; that has a negative impact on the physical or psychological health, development, and identity of the person; and that is the result of gendered power inequities that exploit distinctions between males and females, among males, and among females. Although not exclusive to women and girls, GBV principally affects them across all cultures. Violence may be physical, verbal, sexual, psychological, economic, or sociocultural. Categories of perpetrators may include family members, community members, and those acting on behalf of or in proportion to the disregard of cultural, religious, state, or intrastate institutions.

Physical abuse is abuse involving contact intended to cause feelings of intimidation, pain, injury, or other physical suffering or bodily harm. Sexual abuse is any situation in which force or threat is used to obtain participation in unwanted sexual activity. Coercing a person to engage in sexual activity against his or her will, even if that person is a spouse or intimate partner with whom consensual sex has occurred, is an act of aggression and violence. Sexual abuse can also be an attempted or completed sex act with a person who is unable to understand the nature or condition of the act, unable to decline participation, or unable to communicate unwillingness to engage in the sexual act, for instance, because of underage immaturity, illness, disability, the influence of alcohol or other drugs, or intimidation or pressure.

Domestic violence is defined as a pattern of abusive behaviour by one partner against another in an intimate relationship such as marriage, dating, family, or cohabitation. It has many forms, including physical aggression or assault (hitting, kicking, biting, shoving, restraining, slapping, throwing objects, or deprivation). The violence is inflicted with the intention of humiliating, intimidating, hurting or injuring, and controlling the victim. Very often, the victim is left without recourse to any help and it is well documented that police and law-enforcement agencies are often gender-insensitive, hostile, absent, or dismissive of domestic violence reports. Research has shown that a major factor in helping a victim to establish lasting independence from the abusive partner is her or his ability to get legal assistance.

It is well recognized that SGBV is closely associated with high risk of HIV infection and unless this linkage is acknowledged and seriously addressed, a key driver of HIV infection is not being recognized. While the UN is promoting the three-zero concept (zero new infections, zero deaths from AIDS-related infections, and zero transmission of HIV between mother to child), a fourth zero should be added: that of zero tolerance to all forms of gender- and sexual gender-based violence.

Addressing Violence against Women

> Eliminate gender inequalities and gender-based abuse and
> violence and increase the capacity of women and girls to protect
> themselves from HIV. —*UNAIDS*[71]

There are several ways a church and congregation can respond to address overt and hidden violence against women through the process of mainstreaming of HIV in the programmes of the church. The following are suggestions:

- Actively raise awareness and address sexual inequality, discrimination and harassment within the church through policies, codes of conduct, and systems of accountability.
- Create safe spaces to enable congregation/community members to talk openly and freely. Within these spaces, discuss socially constructed roles and relationships—the norms and practices that shape gender relations, reinforce certain behaviours, and which may affect each other's health, well-being, and, particularly, vulnerability. Do not avoid sensitive topics of sexual diversity because they are controversial, as they are a reality and need to be addressed openly, nonjudgmentally, and in a spirit of unconditional love.
- Advocate trainings around issues of SGBV.
- Develop a crisis-response team who can react immediately and are trained to respond/refer appropriately, compassionately, and to accompany those most in need.
- Be aware of the location of safe houses for survivors of domestic abuse and seek advice on protection issues.
- Ensure confidentiality for survivors and assist them to access the legal protection they require.
- Organize support groups.
- Actively involve boys and men of the church to raise awareness among their peers, whether at school, work, or in recreation places. Support a transforming movement of men who promote gender justice, zero tolerance toward GBV, "not in our name" (zero support for any violence perpetrated by men

toward women), and to stand up for what is morally right. Ensure the basic human rights of girls and women are protected.

- Help rebuild the confidence and self-esteem of those who suffer and have suffered by offering unconditional love, solidarity, and accompaniment.
- Be informed of the complexity and diversity of gender and gender-based violence.
- Network and collaborate and engage with partners including national governments, NGOs, and other faith-based organizations to promote and support gender justice and empowerment programmes.

Example: Church, Family, Relationships, and the HIV and AIDS Programme of the Christian AIDS Task Force (CAT)[72]

This is a gender-justice transformation programme which specifically avoids using the term *gender* to ensure that it does not discourage the participation of men. It is run principally by the Presbyterian churches in a poor peri-urban area with largely migrants and in a rural area, steeped in traditional practices, in a remote part of southern Zimbabwe.

A comprehensive baseline survey was first undertaken to determine whether or not churches in these areas were experiencing gender-related problems and whether or not there was a desire to address the issues. The survey identified many such problems, including multiple concurrent sexual partners, lack of empowerment of women, general family-relationship breakdowns, skepticism about marriage, and poor communication skills between the genders and generations. The survey also identified many negative cultural practices justified as "biblical truths."

The programme they have developed aims at challenging attitudes toward gender relationships, initially through targeting church leaders on gender equality and working together with the community. Gender was mainstreamed into all the activities of CAT. The programme involves men, women, and people living with HIV and seeks to strengthen relationships between the church and broader community. Included in the programme are skills training in communication problems, discussions on abusive relationships, basic counselling for couples, values, and realizing dreams. A sound basis in HIV knowledge has also been introduced.

The programme has proven to be very successful, with numerous testimonies of significant change in gender relationships and understanding of each other. For many women, the changes have included a life free of violence, increased decision-making powers, and protection of many of their rights which had previously been ignored or violated.

8.13 Orphans and Vulnerable Children

> Let the little children come to me, and do not hinder them, for
> the kingdom of heaven belongs to such as these.
> —*Matthew 19:13-14*

> Children have been the missing face of the AIDS pandemic. An
> estimated 15 million children around the world have lost one or
> both parents to AIDS. These children need support, education
> and protection. —*Ann Veneman*[73]

Orphans and vulnerable children represent one of the greatest challenges of the HIV epidemic. The sheer numbers of children affected are unprecedented in history and will continue to rise until a universally accessible cure for HIV is found. The complexity of their needs and the long-term commitment required means that orphans and vulnerable children cannot be tagged onto some other programme such as "care" or "counselling and psychosocial support." Further-more, the age range of children affected means that no one solution fits all. We cannot ignore these statistics, realizing they represent children—the vulnerable of society. Orphan care and support is in itself an HIV preventative strategy. They need their own stand-alone programme, which is fully comprehensive.[74] There is no doubt that in human development and financial terms, the cost of care now will be less than the price society will ultimately pay for the neglect of these children left to a life on the streets, in the bush, or in institutions.[75]

For many churches across Africa, the challenge of orphans is one of the most pressing and distressing challenges and many churches are at a real loss at what to do. Some have introduced programmes of support, which include the provision of some of the basic necessities such as school fees, feeding schemes, clothing, and assistance with accessing legal documents such as birth certificates. More comprehensive programmes include support for the extended family or ensuring appropriate guardianship; psychosocial support; health care including HIV awareness and supporting access to appropriate treatment if individuals are HIV-positive; and child-empowerment programmes. Many churches have been involved in the provision of institutionalized care but the sheer magnitude of the numbers needing care requires a more sustainable, culturally sensitive and appropriate care, without sibling separation, in an environment where they can learn their culture firsthand. This is best done through providing the required support where necessary but focusing on strengthening the coping capacities of families and communities to respond to children orphaned and made vulnerable. Building broad collaboration among key stakeholders in all sectors ensures that the process of response is comprehensive and sustainable and that the children become everyone's responsibility. At the same time, there is need to appreciate that children have strengths and resilience and need also to be involved as active participants in decisions that affect them. While it is important to ensure that these children have their rights respected and realized; that they are afforded proper child protection and receive the same opportunities as their unaffected peers; that they have opportunity to *be* children, perhaps the most important aspect is to empower the children.

Empowerment can be conceptualized as *the ability to make choices and make changes.* In order to break the cycle of their being victims of circumstances, and to give them a light at the end of the tunnel in all the varied hardships they face as a consequence of their circumstances, empowerment is the key. It moves beyond ensuring needs are met to enabling them to believe in a future where they can meet their own needs and believe in themselves.

Examples: Anglican Church's Fikelela Children's Centre[76]

Based in Khayelitsha, Cape Town, the Children's Centre currently cares for 26 orphaned, abandoned, vulnerable, neglected, or HIV-positive children. It was started by the Anglican Church in response to the dire situation of these children and is now registered with social services. These children find protection, nutrition, care, support, medical treatment, and love. They remain in care while an alternative, more permanent solution is found for them within the community.

The *Giving Hope* Empowerment Methodology of Church World Service

Background. The *Giving Hope* empowerment methodology evolved over a period of three years (2003–2005), as the international organization Church World Service worked in conjunction with partners across East Africa. It grew out of the partners' search for new ways to address the dilemma of growing numbers of orphans and vulnerable children emerging from both the growing impact of HIV and AIDS and from the conflicts in the Great Lakes region.

Traditionally, orphans would be cared for within the extended family system but the sheer numbers of orphans have overwhelmed and overstretched the time-honoured system, with increasing numbers of children falling through this safety net, leading to the emergence of child-headed households. Adolescents and young adults from about 12 to 24 years of age, referred to as youth caregivers, are shouldering, sometimes exclusively, the primary care responsibilities for their younger siblings and, often times, ailing adults.

The *Giving Hope* asset-based empowerment methodology presents an alternative approach to the more common responses of seeking to meet the needs of these children. It redirects attention from *needs*, to instead focus and respond to youth's *assets*—ideas, skills, resilience, and renewed relationships. The methodology builds upon the significant strengths that youth caregivers and their households possess by:

1. Restoring relationships, structures, and routines in youth caregivers' lives.

2. Recognizing and reinforcing youth caregivers' existing assets: their existing knowledge, skills, resources, resilience, and newly restored relationships.

Youth Caregiver Outcomes of Asset-based Empowerment. The *Giving Hope* methodology has led to four key outcomes. These have been an improvement in youth caregivers' sense of self, belonging, power, and collective responsibility:

1. *Sense of Self.* Typified through youth caregivers' creation of a *dream,* a personal reflection process, these dreams have restored youth's sense of self, purpose, optimism, vision, and hope for the future and also become the goals that they work to realize.

2. *Sense of Belonging.* Youth working-group members have become like extended family members for youth caregivers and their households, with each group having an adult mentor who provides moral support.

3. *Sense of Power.* This has been achieved through youth caregivers' participation in *livelihood activities* that contribute to youth working-group savings accounts, as well as future lending activities to facilitate the realization of youth caregiver dreams. Youth have accessed group funds to engage in skill training and launch small businesses.

4. *Sense of Collective Responsibility.* Youth have reached out to assist and accompany other youth caregivers regularly. Observed examples of youth outreach include the mentoring of another youth to leave the streets and join their youth working group, educating peers in HIV prevention, and serving on community development committees.

Benchmarks on Competence: Orphans and Vulnerable Children

> Don't steal the land of defenseless orphans by moving the ancient boundary markers. —*Proverbs 23:10*

> He gives justice to orphans and widows. He shows love to the foreigners living among you and gives them food and clothing.
> —*Deuteronomy 10:18*

1. Do we have special programmes addressing the needs of vulnerable children? These include:
- Provision of shelter
- Protection against exploitation, violence, and sexual abuse
- Support in documentation/identity papers and legal assistance
- Educational support
- Health and nutritional support
- Safe water and sanitation access
- Psycho-social support
- Work for their empowerment, development of life skills, and long-term future

2. Have we made a concerted effort to strengthen the skills and caring capacity of the primary social safety net of orphans and vulnerable children—the families and communities?

3. Are parents who are living with HIV encouraged to write wills and provide a succession plan for their children?

4. Have we built on children and young people's resilience and increased their capacity to meet their own needs through facilitating the above?

8.14 Ecumenism and Interfaith Collaboration

Meaningful and respectful cooperation with other Christian denominations and with other faiths is a way of addressing HIV as it affects all our communities. Having a common venue, such as ministers' fraternal meetings, provides an opportunity to listen to others' experiences and to share. Ecumenical services provide opportunity to address HIV in a collaborative way and a means of demonstrating a unified stand against stigma and discrimination and acknowledging the common challenge of HIV in our families and in our communities.

Some church leaders are cautious about entering into networks with other agencies which advocate HIV-prevention techniques that may be considered to be contrary to the church's moral teaching. It should be possible to identify different ethical approaches and explore ways of complementing rather than confronting. There are plenty of success stories.

Churches can collaborate with organizations that provide technical support and thus better document and evaluate their work. This will enhance credibility and lessons learned and enable scaling-up of successful strategies.

In some countries the government and the UN agencies do not like dealing with multiple faiths over the issue of HIV and AIDS. They require a common voice. Hence, Christian AIDS networks and interfaith coalitions have been developed, demonstrating the possibilities of working together and having a strong voice in advocating for the rights of people living with HIV and access to treatment and services.

All collaboration and partnerships, particularly between the government sector, multilateral and bilateral agencies/donors, and implementing agencies (civil society, NGOs, and FBOs) require mutual respect and balance. Other factors, often more hidden, that limit networking involve issues such as problems with power sharing, guilt at having HIV as a reality within the church, and competition for funding from the same donors.[77]

Example: Zambia Interfaith Networking Group on HIV/AIDS (ZINGO)

Organizational profile. In 1997 the Zambia Interfaith Networking Group on HIV/AIDS (ZINGO) was established to provide leadership in the faith response to the rising challenges of HIV and AIDS. The mandate is to coordinate, network, build competencies, and mobilize technical and material resources for religious communities willing to become more involved in HIV and AIDS prevention, care, and intervention support. ZINGO consists of the four major Christian umbrella bodies in Zambia, namely the Christian Council of Zambia (CCZ), the Evangelical Fellowship of Zambia (EFZ), the Independent Churches of Zambia (ICOZ), and the Zambia Episcopal Conference (ZEC), along with the Islamic Council of Zambia and the Baha'i and Hindu communities in Zambia. Together these faith mother bodies share a common vision of an interfaith community that is free from the threat of HIV and AIDS, and to realize the mandate, they have partnered with many key stakeholders in the country.

Prevention. ZINGO supports programmes for in- and out-of-school youths with HIV and AIDS behavior-change messages. It reaches out to minors in sex work with behavior-change messages and helps them to reintegrate into the school system as part of a reform process. ZINGO has also entered into partnership with Local Partners Capacity Building Programme (LPCB), with the agreement to build the capacity of partner organizations implementing prevention activities.

In the village of Musokotwane in Kazungula, ZINGO is working with young single mothers who dropped out of school due to unwanted pregnancies to reintegrate them into the school system. ZINGO is also assisting the same young single mothers with economic and livelihood opportunities to sustain their lives and the lives of their babies as part of a support to sustain behavior change and promote good health.

In Lusaka, ZINGO is working with FBOs in a pilot project that is aimed at bringing counselling and testing services and promotion of sexual reproductive health rights to the local congregational level as part of a strategy to the promotion of sexual health.

Treatment care and support. In the area of treatment, care, and support, ZINGO is working with its implementing FBO partners to provide care and support to people living with HIV and other vulnerable members of society. This support includes palliative care, psycho-social support, provision of nutrition (through an innovative and sustainable approach of encouraging nutritional gardens) to the sick, and referral of cases to specialized health clinics. Recently and through partnership with the Global Fund, ZINGO's members have started to integrate care and support of TB in their HIV and AIDS home-care programmes in order to address the burden of co-infection and promote quality care and support for people living with HIV.

Home-based care. The high prevalence of HIV-related illnesses in Zambia has seriously overburdened the health-care system at all levels, hence the need to have well-organized, efficient, and fully equipped home-based care groups that would complement government efforts.

ZINGO, as an interfaith coordinating body, resolved to coordinate the efforts of home-based care groups within parishes, mosques, and local congregations in the theme of providing care and support to people living with HIV. ZINGO believes that supporting the well-being of people living with HIV is important from a practical perspective and crucial from a human rights perspective. ZINGO also believes that home-based care services are critical in reducing the burden on the health system while leading to improvement in the quality of life.

Impact mitigation. In the area of impact mitigation, ZINGO is involved in a fatherhood and parenthood project to encourage positive parenting that will reduce children's vulnerabilities to HIV and AIDS. ZINGO is also working with its implementing FBO partners to integrate a child-rights approach in child programming so as to ensure comprehensive and sustainable solutions and responses to issues regarding children. Similarly, and as part of providing psycho-social support to vulnerable children, ZINGO is working with a number of faith-based community schools to introduce sporting activities through its "Kicking AIDS Out" Project.

Benchmarks on Competence: Ecumenism and Interfaith Cooperation
Meaningful and respectful cooperation with other Christian denominations and with other faiths. Has HIV been addressed:
1. In ecumenical church services?
2. In collaborative action (both interdenominational and interreligious)?
3. Do we have venues to listen to each other's experiences?

Stewardship of Time, Talents, Finances, and Resources

Much will be required of the person entrusted with much, and still more will be demanded of the person entrusted with even more.
—*Luke 12:48*

Stewardship is a way of life that is expected of Christians, based on many scriptural references in both the Old and New Testaments. It is an expression of gratitude to God and reminds us that we are entrusted with assets and are not the owners of them. We have gifts of time, talents, skills, and resources that can be shared as an expression of our love and gratitude to God as well as a means of strengthening and furthering the good news and hope of the gospel.

In the same way, our churches and faith institutions must be accountable to the community for the way in which the church utilizes the gifts entrusted to it.

Where donor funds have been accessed to support programmes it is essential that there be full and transparent accountability for these funds. "All partners—funders, implementers, those accessing services, technical support providers, policy makers, advocates—must be accountable to each other. Accountability and transparency are not for some actors and organizations only: They must apply to all who are engaged, from the global to the individual level."[1]

In order to mainstream HIV and to be able to effectively and sustainably respond to the many diverse needs created by this epidemic, the church must maximally utilize the many resources it already has in terms of structures, skills, talents, and volunteers within the church, as well as the extensive networks and linkages from grassroots to the international community. It requires a dedicated budget line and commitment to raise additional resources to meet emerging needs.

All these resources need to be utilized with maximum transparency and accountability and the activities undertaken should be appropriate and timely, have minimal wastage, and be held to a high standard.

5

Benchmarks on Competence: Stewardship of Finances and Resources

The congregation, being aware of and mobilizing the resources that are available within the community, attempting to mobilize additional resources needed to serve better, and being accountable to all concerned, asks:

1. Is there a person mandated to follow through on the issue of HIV within the congregation?

2. Do we utilize available structures of our church for our HIV-related work (structures could mean schools, church, clinics, and hospital)?

3. Is there a budget line devoted to HIV in the finances of the congregation?

4. Do we mobilize financial resources for HIV from within the congregation?

5. Do we receive external funding for our programmes?

6. Do we document what we do and communicate to all concerned?

7. Are there mechanisms which ensure that we are accountable to each other and to the people we serve and receive resources from (boards, committees, audited and publicized financial reports)?

Section 10
Monitoring, Evaluation, and Knowledge Sharing

Are we doing the right thing and are we doing it right? A project is seen as being successfully mainstreamed if it:

- Reaches its core business objectives;
- Removes barriers and enables people living with HIV and affected people to participate in and derive benefits from the project activities;
- Minimizes the potential risk of HIV transmission and the impacts of HIV on beneficiary groups, staff, and volunteers;
- Enables or facilitates linkages to appropriate services;
- Builds the capacity for analysis and intervention at all levels;
- Generates and uses evidence to improve our own work and influence the policy and practice environment in which we work.[1]

There is need for consistent documentation and monitoring and evaluation as a confirmatory and a learning process and for sharing knowledge and expertise between partner churches and organizations. Mainstreaming is aimed at making practical and plausible changes as appropriate, both internally and externally. It is crucial to monitor progress actively. Policies can set out excellent ideas, but they may then be ignored or misapplied. Ongoing monitoring of the application of the policies, and their effects, provides the opportunity to modify and improve both policies and practice. In the same way, planned activities and changes need to be monitored, assessed, and revised as necessary.[2]

How the church plans to monitor and evaluate the programmes should be considered from early on, as should the capacity requirements. It is of value to ensure that data collected is disaggregated by sex, age, and other relevant diversity factors as it in turn ensures that gender and sexuality is mainstreamed into the programmes and that they do not get buried.

It is not always easy to measure changes as the activities are geared to addressing underlying causes of HIV at all levels. Monitoring tracks what happened (outcome monitoring) while evaluation (impact monitoring) assesses the value, that is, the changes observed and whether the programme is making a difference.

It is not usually possible to attribute all impacts to one programme or intervention as it is more likely to be the result of many interventions over time. Your intervention may just be a catalyst to the overall process of change. It is best to describe what is observed in the outcomes and how these outcomes relate to the impact experienced.

10.1 Indicators

Indicators represent ways to measure how successful something has been and should link well with the aim, objective, and those with whom you work—the audience. Indicators are observable and measurable "milestones" toward an outcome target.[3] There are principally two types of measures: *quantitative* and *qualitative*.

Quantitative measurement concerns numbers—for example, the number of people trained, the number of people in a support group, and the like. They are exact but measure only one narrow aspect, which may or may not be indicative of reaching overall objectives.

Qualitative measurement refers to recording "descriptive," "narrative," "open questions" (what has changed?) responses. They are difficult to summarize in progress reports but may help to spot unexpected results and underlying reasons, whether positive or negative.[4]

10.2 Outcome Monitoring

Outcome monitoring is done to assess what actually happened—the immediate or midterm effects of programmes and the mainstreaming process, compared against objectives. Outcome focuses on effectiveness of the programme activities undertaken. Key questions:

- To what extent and how have we achieved the objective?
- Why have we achieved something?
- How have we collaborated with other stakeholders?

10.3 Impact Monitoring

Impact monitoring is done to assess long-term effects and changes on beneficiaries, affected groups, and institutions and the value of those changes. Has the programme made any difference in the lives of the people we serve and with whom we work? Key questions:

- Does it make sense?
- Are the programme strategies and objectives relevant?
- Are we doing the right things?
- Are there changes in terms of determinants/vulnerabilities and impact mitigation?

10.4 Knowledge Sharing

By sharing knowledge, we learn from our own activities and we learn from others. It is a strengthening process and is vital if we are serious about making a difference in the lives of the people and the community served by the church.

Sharing best practices and learning from others helps to confirm the validity of our responses or provides the evidence to instigate changes in our activities and thus formulate more effective responses. This is the ultimate aim of all responses to HIV: effectively and sustainably to make a difference. For churches, however, there is an added dimension to all we do and seek to do. The ultimate aim of all our efforts is the restoration of hope and dignity to all who are infected and all who are affected by HIV.

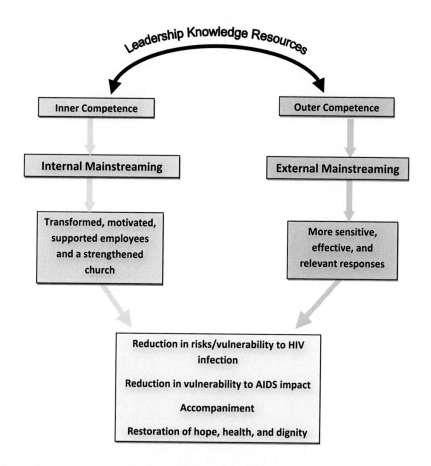

CONCLUSION

Jesus wept. —*John 11:35*

It is now some 30 years since AIDS became a reality in our lives and the virus, HIV, became a real threat to individuals, families, communities, and society as a whole. It is a virus which has caused untold suffering, stripping away the health and future of millions, lowering life expectancy, and threatening to reverse economic gains in many countries, leaving a swath of devastation in its path, including millions of orphans. No country has been unaffected. More than any other global catastrophe, it has brought different people together to seek common solutions which would mitigate the impact and prevent the ongoing transmission of the virus.

Today we have hope as we look toward the possibility of an AIDS-free generation, while we continue to seek a cure so we ultimately also have *an HIV-free* generation. Yet even while treatment is available to reduce the viral load and maintain a healthy immune system, the sad reality is that not everyone who needs such care and treatment is accessing it and the numbers of new infections in many countries still outpace the numbers accessing life-saving therapy. Stigma and discrimination, prejudice and judgment, indifference and denial, intolerance and rejection, all still remain rooted in our hearts and in our actions, whether knowingly or not.

We live in a world which has increasingly become secularized and focused on the individual. It is a "quick-fix" society, with less sense of responsibility, commitment, or care for the other than perhaps at any other time in our history. At the same time, this devastating HIV has challenged us in so many different ways as it has exposed injustices, "flaws and cracks," in our societies, in our socioeconomic disparities, in gender norms, traditions, cultures, and especially in our accepted theologies. It has thrown the spotlight on the many inequities and inequalities that characterize our societies and service deliveries, and it has forced us to break the silence on the sexual and gender-based violence that is so pervasive in our societies—from domestic violence and abuse on one extreme to state-sponsored rape as a form of political oppression or war at the other extreme. It has raised our awareness on the skewed health-service availability, the immorality of pharmaceutical patents in the face of massive numbers of avoidable deaths, and a host of other challenges so prevalent in today's world.

HIV and its consequences will be with us for a long time to come. We are all vulnerable to its impact, and many of us, as well as those we love, are also at risk of infection. To acknowledge and personalize the risks that HIV poses brings an inner transformation to our attitudes and approach to HIV. Facing these issues in an open and honest manner adds credibility and authenticity to any subsequent response. As we respond to HIV in a holistic manner, we are also responding to the many key drivers of this epidemic, which are detrimental flaws in our society that we have complacently accepted or chosen to ignore. HIV is the catalyst to changing our attitudes and challenging us not only to respond to the devastating condition of HIV, but also to seek healing and wholeness for our society in every aspect.

This book has sought to provide guidelines for translating the principles of inner and outer competence into practice within our own lives, in our families, and in every aspect of the life of the church. Not only do we seek to prevent the ongoing transmission of the virus and mitigate its impact, but we also seek to restore dignity and hope to ourselves and to those amongst us who are affected and suffering under the burden of HIV. In the process, may we find again the compassion which characterized the unconditional love of our Lord.

By internally mainstreaming HIV competence in the church (the inner domain), all those who work in and for the church should feel recognized and supported and find both inner transformation and renewed motivation. As HIV competence is mainstreamed in the various activities and programmes of the church (the outer domain), with the full involvement of people concerned as partners, the responses are likely to be more sensitive, effective, relevant, caring, and compassionate. The combined effect should be a greater awareness of the risks of HIV infection and an enhanced ability to deal with both the risks and vulnerability to infection. Mitigation against the impact can thus be more relevant. The compassionate, knowledgeable accompaniment of those most affected by HIV can restore hope, health, and dignity, for though "medicines may give us a *means* to live; faith gives us a *reason* to live."[1]

Ultimately, not only will the church be responding competently to *HIV* but also to so many of the deep-seated, scarring problems in society which undermine our lives as individuals, our relationships, and our societies.

It is my fervent prayer that this be so.

> May our Lord Jesus Christ Himself and God our Father, who loved us and by His grace gave us eternal encouragement and good hope, encourage your hearts and strengthen you in every good deed and word. —*2 Thessalonians 2:16*

Benchmarks

The following benchmarks are used throughout the preceding text and are drawn from *Beacons of Hope: HIV Competent Churches—A Framework for Action* (Geneva: WCC Publications, 2008). They are offered here in full, with only minor edits.

HIV-Competent Church: Benchmarks and Self-Assessment Tool

An HIV-competent church is one that recognizes and accepts the imperatives of HIV to itself and communities; has the knowledge, willingness, and experience to respond in an inclusive, effective, and prophetic manner that reflects the fruits of a Spirit-filled congregation. The response of the HIV-competent church to the pandemic is characterized by love, joy, peace, patience, kindness, goodness, gentleness, faithfulness, and self-control (Galatians 5:22-23).

We can ask ourselves: Is my church HIV-competent? Do you want to find out?

Good intentions, policies, and plans are crucial but are incomplete without sustained action that follows consistently to ensure societal transformation and life-enhancing responses. A good tree is recognized by its good fruits (Matthew 7:20).

Our response as individuals and as a congregation to the crisis the world faces in the form of HIV contributes to how we are defined as communities and recognized as followers of our Lord Jesus Christ.

> "A new command I give you: Love one another. As I have loved you, so you must love one another. By this all men will know that you are my disciples, if you love one another." —John 13:34-35

In the context of HIV, we as people of faith have the responsibility to work to the highest possible standard. To this end, there is a tremendous need for us to truthfully assess the quantum and the quality of our responses. This will not only help us to identify our contributions, but will help us to identify our weaknesses and strengths, and to monitor our effectiveness as an HIV-competent church. The self-assessment tool that is given below has been developed by church workers and theologians who have been deeply involved in the churches' work to overcome HIV. It is hoped that this assessment tool will be used by groups, as a community activity for self-assessment and peer review.

If we do not have policies in place, let us create them in a participatory manner. If we have policies, let us ensure that we implement them as a church or church-related organization. Let us periodically assess ourselves to ensure that our efforts are relevant, effective, and sustained.

A. Pastoral care
Care in the context of our own faith that is edifying and supportive.
Does my church have:

1. Systems that ensure home visits when people are sick, including possibility of individual counselling for those among us who are HIV+? *(0 for none, 1 indicating basic functioning system, 2 indicating a good system, 3 indicating excellent)*

2. Systems such as area fellowships and accompaniment programmes that provide support for affected families? *(0 for none, 1 indicating basic functioning system, 2 indicating a good system, 3 indicating excellent)*

3. Marriage-enhancement programmes? *(0 for no, 2 indicating yes)*

4. Pre- and post-marriage counselling? *(0 for no, 2 indicating yes)*

5. Do we minister to the needs of widows, widowers, and single parents? *(0 for no, 2 indicating yes)*

6. Safe spaces/forums for addressing diverse issues such as domestic violence and incest *(0 for none, 1 indicating basic functioning system, 2 indicating a good system, 3 indicating excellent)*

B. Homilies/preaching
The spoken word and the writing we commit on paper in the place of worship and in the context of worship, as leaders, clergy, and laity.

1. How often do we hear HIV being addressed in sermons? *(0 for none, 1 indicating one event, 2 indicating 2, 3 indicating 3, 5 more than 3)*

2. What is the quality of the message? *(-2 for stigmatizing, 0 for poor, 2 indicating good, 4 for inspiring/thought provoking)*

3. Are our leaders knowledgeable and trained on the issue? *(0 for no, 1 indicating adequate, 2 indicating good level)*

4. Have there been specific publications/periodicals/newsletters addressing HIV? *(0 for none, 2 indicating one, 4 indicating 2, 6 indicating more than 3)*

5. Is the issue addressed in other publications/periodicals/newsletters? *(0 for none, 1 indicating one, 2 indicating 2, 3 indicating more than 3, and 4 indicating 4 or more)*

C. Liturgy
Worship which includes silence, contemplation, words, songs, dances, and practices that are used to communicate with God in fellowship and in solitude.

1. Do we have HIV-specific liturgies for funerals, marriages, confirmation? *(0 for no, 2 indicating yes)*

2. Have our routine liturgies incorporated and addressed HIV? *(0 for no, 2 indicating yes)*

3. Do we celebrate healing services/liturgies? *(0 for no, 2 indicating yes)*

4. Do we say special prayers for those of us who are living with HIV and affected by it? *(0 for no, 2 indicating yes)*

D. Faith formation and moral education
Formation that that helps us to incorporate the Christian values into our daily lives.
Have we incorporated HIV (in the form of change in curriculum, addition of workshops and seminars) in our:

1. Sunday schools? *(0 for no, 2 indicating yes)*

2. Youth groups? *(0 for no, 2 indicating yes)*

3. Women's fellowships? *(0 for no, 2 indicating yes)*

4. Men's fellowships? *(0 for no, 2 indicating yes)*

5. The whole congregation? *(0 for no, 2 indicating yes)*

E. Ecumenism and interfaith cooperation
Meaningful and respectful cooperation with other Christian denominations and with other faiths.
Has HIV been addressed in:

1. Ecumenical church services? *(0 for none, 2 indicating one event, 4 indicating 2, 6 indicating more than 2)*

2. Collaborative action? (both interdenominational and interreligious) *(0 for none, 2 indicating one event, 4 indicating 2, 6 indicating more than 2)*

3. Do we have venues to listen to each other's experiences? *(0 for no, 2 indicating one event, 4 indicating 2, 6 indicating more than 2)*

F. Meaningful participation of those among us who are HIV+

1. How many of us are openly positive in our church? *(0 for none, 2 indicating one member, 4 indicating 2, 6 indicating more than 2)*

2. How many of our leaders are openly positive? *(0 for none, 2 indicating one leader, 4 indicating 2, 6 indicating more than 2)*

3. Do we have a workplace policy that is conducive to those among us who are HIV+? *(0 for none, 1 for one being developed, 3 for adopted)*

4. Are those among us who are HIV+ part of committees in our church? *(0 none, 3 for membership in one committee, 6 for more than one committee)*

5. Do those among us who are positive feel welcomed and embraced in the congregation? *(-2 for feeling stigmatized, 0 for mixed, 1 marginally good, 2 good, 3 very good)*

6. Do we have retreats or capacity-building programmes for those among us who are positive? *(0 for none, 2 indicating one or more programmes)*

G. Prevention
Addressing prevention of HIV in a holistic manner and making us less vulnerable.

1. Is human sexuality addressed in a sound, forthright, and scientific manner and addressed to different age groups? *(0 for no, 1 marginally good, 2 good, 3 very good)*

2. Do we discuss the social factors that can make us vulnerable to HIV? *(0 for no, 1 for marginally good discussions, 2 for good discussions, 3 very good discussions)*

3. Do we deal with cultural practices within our own society that enhance our vulnerability or protect us? *(0 for no, 1 marginally dealing with cultural practices, 2 good, 3 very good)*

4. Do we reach out to those among us who are vulnerable or in our communities or do we behave as if such a population does not exist? *(0 for no, 1 marginally affirming, 2 affirming and reaching out, 4 strongly affirming and reaching out)*

5. In our education and activities on prevention, do we complete our information with scientifically proved and evidence-based methods such as use of condoms, clean needles, and syringes? *(0 for no, 3 for yes)*

H. Care
Caring for those of us in our congregation and in our community who are hurting with HIV.

1. Do we have home-based care programmes? *(0 for no; 2 for first-level care: occasional—once in two weeks or less frequent visits and material support; 4 for second-level care: regular visits—more fortnightly visits and material support; 6 for comprehensive-care programme which includes care, prevention and treatment, and holistic support)*

2. Do we provide nutritional aid? *(0 for no, 2 for yes)*

3. Do we provide legal aid to those among us who are positive or marginalized? *(0 for no, 2 for yes)*

4. Do we see prevention as part of care? *(0 for no, 2 for yes)*

I. Vulnerable children
Let the little children come to me, and do not hinder them, for the kingdom of heaven belongs to such as these. (Matthew 19:13-14)

Don't steal the land of defenseless orphans by moving the ancient boundary markers. (Proverbs 23:10)

He gives justice to orphans and widows. He shows love to the foreigners living among you and gives them food and clothing. (Deuteronomy 10:18)

Do we have special programmes addressing the needs of vulnerable children?

1. Provision of shelter *(0 for no, 2 for yes)*

2. Protection against exploitation and sexual abuse *(0 for no, 2 for yes)*

3. Support in documentation/identity papers and legal assistance? *(0 for no, 2 for yes)*

4. Educational support? *(0 for no, 2 for yes)*

5. Nutritional support? *(0 for no, 2 for yes)*

6. Psycho-social support? *(0 for no, 2 for yes)*

7. Work for the empowerment and long-term future? *(0 for no, 2 for yes)*

J. Treatment
The congregation facilitating and sustaining the access to life-giving treatment.

1. We as a community take steps to promote treatment literacy—like giving information, conducting seminars/workshops, and training of congregation members *(0 for no, 1 for satisfactory actions, 2 for good actions)*

2. Do we know where we can refer pregnant women and their spouses to be screened and to benefit from the prevention of parent-to-child transmission of HIV and would we advise them to utilize the service? *(0 for no, 2 for yes)*

3. Involved in dispensing of medicines/facilitates buddy programme (individuals who are trained and committed to accompany a person in need)? *(0 for no, 1 for satisfactory actions, 2 for good actions)*

4. Provides treatment of opportunistic infections and ARV *(0 for no, 1 for satisfactory programmes, 2 for good programmes)*

K. Counselling and testing

Opportunities within our community's own sacred space to test for HIV in a supportive, confidential, and secure manner.

1. Do our leaders and members know where testing is being done? *(0 for no, 1 for yes)*

2. Is the congregation connected to and can refer members to testing facilities? *(0 for no, 1 for yes)*

3. Do we have facilities within our own structures for testing? *(0 for no, 1 for yes)*

4. Do we maintain confidentiality? *(0 for no, 1 for yes)*

5. Can discordant couples (when one partner is HIV+ and the other is negative) who are among us get sound advice and support from our congregation? *(0 for no, 1 for yes)*

L. Stewardship of finances and resources

The congregation being aware of and mobilizing the resources that are available within the community, attempting to mobilize additional resources needed to serve better, and being accountable to all concerned.

1. Is there a person mandated to follow through on the issue of HIV within the congregation? *(0 for no, 1 for a person is held responsible, 2 for a person is both held responsible and has a clear-cut programme)*

2. Do we utilize available structures of our church for our HIV-related work (structures could mean schools, church, clinics, and hospitals)? *(0 for no, 1 for satisfactory use of facilities, 2 for good use of facilities)*

3. Is there a budget line devoted to HIV in the finances of the congregation? *(0 for no, 1 for yes)*

4. Do we mobilize financial resources for HIV from within the congregation? *(0 for no, 1 for yes)*

5. Do we receive external funding for our programmes? *(0 for no, 1 for yes)*

6. Do we document what we do and communicate to all concerned? *(0 for no, 1 for yes)*

7. Are there mechanisms which ensure that we are accountable to each other and to the people we serve and receive resources from (boards, committees, audited and publicized financial reports)? *(0 for no, 3 for yes)*

NOTES

Introduction

1. United Nations, "Political Declaration on HIV/AIDS: Intensifying our Efforts to Eliminate HIV/AIDS," 8 July 2011, Resolution 65/277, 20110610_UN_A-RES-65-277_en.pdf.

2. Referring to HIV alone is now the preferred option in documentation, unless one is specifically referring to AIDS; however, within this handbook there will be reference to HIV *and* AIDS, as the church is also dealing with impacts of AIDS and end-of-life issues.

3. Examples from the World Council of Churches Ecumenical HIV and AIDS Initiative in Africa (EHAIA) documents include: Musa Dube, ed., *HIV/AIDS Curriculum for Theological Institutions* (in English, French, Spanish and Portuguese; 2003); Ezra Chitando, *Mainstreaming HIV and AIDS in Theological Education: Experiences and Explorations* (2008); Musa Dube, series editor, *HIV and AIDS Curriculum for Theological Education by Extension in Africa & 10 HIV and AIDS Modules* (2007).

4. Archbishop Anastasios of Tirana and Durres, Orthodox primate of Albania and a WCC president, on the significance of mission in the lives of the churches; *WCC News*, 2012.

5. Church staff: all employed staff inclusive of clergy, office bearers, and volunteers; i.e., all actively doing and involved in service provision and ministry.

6. UNAIDS/GTZ, *Mainstreaming HIV/AIDS: A Conceptual Framework and Implementation Principles* (June 2002), http://www.afronets.org/files/mainstream.pdf.

7. Mlisana Koleka, associate professor and head of the medical microbiology department at the University KwaZulu-Natal and NHLS, in a message to delegates at the 6th South Africa AIDS Conference, 2013, http://kaliwise.com/2013/06/message-from-the-sa-aids-conference-chair-prof-koleka-mlisana.

Section 1. Why This Handbook?

1. Sue Parry, *Beacons of Hope: HIV Competent Churches—A Framework for Action* (Geneva: WCC Publications, 2008).

Section 2. The Scope of the HIV and AIDS Epidemic Today

1. United Nations General Assembly, "Political Declaration on HIV and AIDS: Intensifying our Efforts to Eliminate HIV and AIDS," Resolution 65/277, 8 July 2011, http://www.unaids.org/en/aboutunaids/unitednationsdeclarationsandgoals/2011highlevelmeetingonaids/.

2. Michel Sidibé, "Introduction: Our Ambitious Vision," in *AIDS at 30: Nations at the Crossroads* (New York: UNAIDS, 2011), 11.

3. Adapted from the UNAIDS Progress Report 2011, *Global HIV/AIDS Response: Epidemic Update and Health Sector Progress towards Universal Access*, http://www.unaids.org/en/resources/publications/2011/name,64437,en.asp .

4. Peter Piot, "Thirty Years Response to HIV and AIDS: Situation and Response Trends in Africa," plenary presentation, ICASA 2011, Addis Ababa, Ethiopia, 5 December 2011.

5. UNAIDS Progress Report, *Global HIV/AIDS Response*, 5.

6. Michel Sidibé, "Shaping the Future We Want," in *Together We Will End AIDS*, UNAIDS 2012 report, 12, http://www.unaids.org/en/resources/campaigns/togetherwewillendaids/.

7. Ibid.

8. UNAIDS Progress Report 2011, *Global HIV/AIDS Response*, 172.

9. Hillary Clinton, Plenary presentation, 16th International Conference on AIDS & STIs in Africa (ICASA), Addis Ababa, Ethiopia, 4–8 December 2011.

10. Sue Parry, *Beacons of Hope: HIV Competent Churches—A Framework for Action* (Geneva: WCC Publications, 2008).

11. Parry, *Beacons of Hope*.

12. See "Preying on the 'Weaker' Sex: Political Violence against Women in Zimbabwe," report produced by IDASA (An African Democracy Institute), the International Center for Transitional Justice (ICTJ), and the Harare Research and Advocacy Unit (RAU). November 2010, http://www.kubatana.net/html/archive/women/101126rau2.asp?sector=WOMEN; and "No Hiding Place: Politically Motivated Rape of Women in Zimbabwe," report prepared by the Harare Research and Advocacy Unit (RAU) and the Zimbabwe Association of Doctors for Human Rights (ZADHR), December 2010, http://www.researchandadvocacyunit.org/index.php?option=com_docman&task=doc_details&gid=170&Itemid=90.

13. *Power in Sexual Relationships: An Opening Dialogue among Reproductive Health Professionals* (New York: Population Council, 2001), http://www.popcouncil.org/pdfs/power.pdf.

14. Suzanne Maman, et al., "The Intersections of HIV and Violence: Directions for Future Research and Interventions," *Social Science and Medicine* 50, no. 4 (February 2000): 459–78; Suzanne Maman, et al., "HIV-Positive Women Report More Lifetime Partner Violence: Findings From a Voluntary Counseling and Testing Clinic in Dar es Salaam, Tanzania," *American Journal of Public Health* 92, no. 8 (August 2002): 1331–37.

15. Sue Parry, *Responses of the Faith-Based Organisations to HIV/AIDS in Sub-Saharan Africa* (Geneva: WCC Publications, 2003).
16. Calle Almedal, UNAIDS 2008, 1.

Section 3. Why the Church Should Be Involved in Mainstreaming HIV

1. From Erlinda N. Sentauris and Liza B. Lamis, eds., *Building HIV Competent Churches: Called to Prophesy, Reconcile and Heal* (Hong Kong: Christian Conference of Asia, 2010), 16, http://www.e-alliance.ch/fileadmin/user_upload/docs/Temp/HIV_Resources/WAD_2011/Building_HIV_Competent_Churches.pdf.

2. *Uniting for Universal Access: Overview Brochure on 2011 High Level Meeting on AIDS*, UNAIDS (2010).

3. African Religious Health Assets Programmes (ARHAP), for the World Health Organization (WHO), *Appreciating Assets: The Contribution of Religion to Universal Access in Africa. Mapping, Understanding, Translating, and Engaging Religious Health Assets in Zambia and Lesotho in Support of Universal Access to HIV/AIDS Treatment, Care and Prevention*, October 2006.

4. World Council of Churches, *Facing AIDS: The Challenge, The Churches' Response*, World Council of Churches study document, 1997, http://www.oikoumene.org/en/resources/documents/wcc-programmes/justice-diakonia-and-responsibility-for-creation/ehaia/world-council-of-churches-statements-and-studies/1997-facing-aids-the-challenge-the-churches-response.

5. Professor Ezra Chitando, Theology Consultant, World Council of Churches—Ecumenical HIV and AIDS Initiative in Africa.

6. Michael Czerny, S.J., response to Rev. Robert J. Vitillo's "Pastoral and Theological Challenges of HIV and AIDS," National Seminar for Priests in Ghana, Accra, Ghana, 16–17 June 2004.

Section 4. HIV and AIDS Competence

1. Sue Parry, *Beacons of Hope: HIV Competent Churches—A Framework for Action* (Geneva: WCC Publications, 2008).

2. Anonymous quote, Justa Paz Organization, Maputo, Mozambique.

3. Parry, *Beacons of Hope.*

4. *CABSA Network* 13 (December 2011), article written by Lyn Van Rooyen, Director of CABSA, to Sue Parry.

5. As above.

Section 5. Mainstreaming

1. Based on UNAIDS definition of mainstreaming, in *Mainstreaming HIV and AIDS in Sectors and Programmes: An Implementation Guide for National Responses* (September 2005), http://web.undp.org/hiv/docs/MainstreamingB[1].pdf.

2. UNAIDS/GTZ, *Mainstreaming HIV/AIDS: A Conceptual Framework and Implementation Principles* (June 2002), http://www.afronets.org/files/mainstream.pdf.

3. Adapted from NGO Code of Good Practice, *Self- Assessment Checklist: Main-streaming HIV*, http://www.hivcode.org.

4. Swiss Agency for Development and Cooperation (SADC), *Mainstreaming HIV/AIDS in Practice: Toolkit for Mainstreaming HIV/AIDS*, http://www.eldis.org/go/country-profiles&id=17740&type=Document#.UfgY-VO3IvQ.

5. UNAIDS/GTZ, Bangkok, 2004

6. Adapted from UNAIDS/UNDP/World Bank, *Mainstreaming HIV and AIDS in Sectors and Programmes: An Implementation Guide for National Responses* (September 2005), http://web.undp.org/hiv/docs/MainstreamingB[1].pdf.

7. Ibid.

8. Pope John Paul II, *Laborem Exercens: On Human Work* (Homebush, NSW: St. Pauls Publications, 1981), para. 6.

9. Australian Catholic Commission for Employment Relations, *The Catholic Church as an Employer in Australia Today* (February 2002), http://www.accer.asn.au/index.php?option=come_docman&task=doc_downloaded&gid=64&itemid=41.

10. UNAIDS, et al., *Mainstreaming HIV and AIDS in Sectors and Programmes.*

11. A baseline survey is a cross-sectional survey to provide quantitative informa-tion on the current situation of the people who work in and for the church (Who? What? Where? When? Why? How?) to give a clear picture as to where the impact would be most felt as it relates to the people concerned and to the work of the church.

12. Adapted from Rose Smart, Revised: *HIV/AIDS toolkit for local govern-ment*, The Health Economics and AIDS Research Division (HEARD), USAID and The Policy Project, 2001. See also Helen Elsey and Prisca Kutengule in collaboration with Sue Holden, et al., *HIV/AIDS Mainstreaming: A definition, some experiences and strategies. A resource developed by HIV/AIDS focal points from government sectors and those that have been working on HIV/AIDS main-streaming*, January 2003.

13. Ecumenical Pharmaceutical Network, *HIV & AIDS Treatment Literacy Guide for Church Leaders* (Nairobi: EPN, 2009).

14. Brot für die Welt and Difäm, *HIV & AIDS, Gender, and Domestic Violence: Implications for Policy and Practice* (Stuttgart: Diakonisches Werk der EKD e.V., 2010), www.brot-fur-die-welt.de/fileadmin/mediapool/2_Downloads/Fachinfor-mationen/Dialog/dialog03–hiv-aids.pdf.

15. SADC, *Mainstreaming HIV and AIDS in Practice.*

16. Adapted from Helen Elsey and Prisca Kutengule, et al., "HIV/AIDS Main-streaming: A Definition, Some Experiences and Strategies: A resource developed by HIV/AIDS focal points from government sectors and those that have been working on HIV/AIDS mainstreaming," Southern Africa Regional Poverty Network (January 2003), http://www.sarpn.org/documents/d0000271/index.php.

17. UNAIDS, et al., *Mainstreaming HIV and AIDS in Sectors and Programmes.*

18. ABC stands for: Abstain; Be faithful, Condomize. SAVE stands for S = Safer practices (including ABC, safe blood products, harm reduction, protective measures

gloves, sterile syringes and needles etc; A = Access to correct up-to-date information, services, treatment, care and support, PMTCT and ARVs, orphan support and advocacy; V = voluntary counseling and routine testing access; E = empowerment and education.

19. Adapted from UNAIDS, et al., *Mainstreaming HIV and AIDS in Sectors and Programmes.*

20. "A shoulder to cry on" is a community support system operative in Swaziland, whereby volunteer community persons are given basic psychosocial support training and guidance on when to refer people for additional help, for instance, in cases of rape. Young people have someone independent to turn to for help and a listening ear when they feel threatened or unable to cope.

21. UNAIDS, *Helping Ourselves: Community Responses to AIDS in Swaziland,* Best Practice series, UNAIDS 06.22E, June 2006, http://www.unaids.org/en/ media/unaids/contentassets/dataimport/publications/irc-pub07/jc1259-swaziland- en.pdf.

22. Comment from Louis Chingander, SAfAIDS Executive Director, Harare, Zimbabwe, 2008.

23. Adapted from the Alliance, "NGO Skills Building Session," World AIDS Conference, Vancouver, July 1996, http://www.aidsalliance.org/eng/.

24. Adapted from NGO of Good Practice: Self-Assessment Checklist —Main- streaming HIV, http://www.hivcode.org.

25. Chart inspired by "Mainstreaming HIV/AIDS in Practice—a toolkit with a collection of resources," Swiss Agency for Development (SDC), 2004.

Section 6. Mainstreaming HIV into Theological Institutions

1. EHAIA Impact Study of 2010 (Geneva: WCC Publications, 2010). See http://www.wcc-coe.org and lists of resources available for mainstreaming HIV and AIDS into the curriculum and into theological programmes.

Section 7. Mainstreaming HIV Competence into the Ministry of the Church

1. Aristotle distinguishes between two intellectual virtues: *sophia* and *phronesis. Sophia* (usually translated "wisdom") is the ability to think well about the nature of the world, to discern why the world is the way it is (sometimes equated with science); *sophia* involves deliberation concerning universal truths. *Phronesis* is the capacity to consider the mode of action in order to deliver change, especially to enhance the quality of life.

2. A retreat is a meeting specifically planned to facilitate a group to step back from day-to-day demands and activities for a period of reflection, concentrated discussion, and strategic thinking about specific issues and future plans. In Latin, a "retreat" means to withdraw or to step back.

3. ABC: A–Abstinence before marriage; B–Be faithful in marriage; C– Condomize.

SAVE: (a) Safe Practices (*A+B+C+PMTCT* + *Safe blood, Safe circumcision + Safe injections + Safe microbicides and vaccines research*); (b) Access to treatment (*for OIs, STDs, PEP, PMTCT, Paeditric, & Adult ART*) and nutrition; (c) Voluntary, routine, and stigma-free counseling and testing; (d) Empowerment of children (*school-going age*), youths, women, men, families, communities, and nations vulnerable to preventable and controllable infections, illnesses, and deaths related to and beyond HIV and AIDS.

4. Empowerment is the ability to make informed choices and to be able to make or bring about required changes.

5. Contextual Bible Studies in the era of HIV and AIDS: a methodology to read the Bible through the eyes of HIV and AIDS. It is an approach that revisits well-known and lesser-known biblical passages to understand the context in which the event(s) took place and to find the contextual relevance for the reader today (a particularly powerful tool with gender and violence issues—using the Tamar story). Promoted by the Ujaama Centre, University of KwaZulu Natal, Pietermaritzburg, South Africa.

6. Sr. Joan Chittister, OSB, closing address, Annual Convention of the National Catholic Educational Association, Milwaukee, Wisconsin, 20 April 2001.

7. http://www.equalacess.org.

8. Resources such as: Musa Dube, ed., *Africa Praying: A Handbook on HIV/AIDS Sensitive Sermon Guidelines and Liturgy* (Geneva: WCC Publications, 2003); Robert Igo, OSB, "Making Sense of Suffering," in *A Window into Hope: An Invitation to Faith in the Context of HIV and AIDS* (Geneva: WCC Publications, 2009), 121–44; and many others.

9. Andrew Doupe, *Partnerships between Churches and People Living with HIV/AIDS Organizations* (Geneva: WCC Publications, 2005), http://www.oikoumene.org/en/resources/documents/wcc-programmes/justice-diakonia-and-responsibility-for-creation/health-and-healing/hivaids/wcc-statements-and-studies/partnerships-between-churches-and-people-living-with-hivaids-organizations.

10. Ibid.

11. See n. 5, above.

12. Manoj Kurian, "Safe Spaces: Transforming Faith Communities Consultation," World Council of Churches, Health and Healing Dept. (2012).

Section 8. Specific Areas in the Life and Ministry of the Church for Mainstreaming

1. Canon Dr. Gideon Baguma Byamugisha, personal discussions and correspondence, August 2012.

2. Keith J. White, Haddon Willmer, reflections on Matthew 18, http://www.childtheology.org.

3. Nove Vailaau, *A Theology of Children* (Wellington: Barnardos New Zealand and Royal New Zealand Plunket Society, 2005), 19; summary version by Elizabeth

Clements, 2008; http://www.taha.org.nz/file/documents/pdf/theology_of_children. pdf. The quote in the extract is from Ministry of Education, *Te Whariki: Early childhood curriculum* (Wellington: Learning Medium, 1996), 9.

4. Viva is an international charity, partnering 44 local networks in 24 countries, representing approximately 2,000 members that work with more than 1.1 million children at risk. Instead of starting new projects, Viva equips the existing work being done by community organizations, NGOs, and churches worldwide, encouraging them to support each other, collaborate, learn, and share resources. This information is used with permission.

5. Reported by an organization called CRANE (Children at Risk Action Network) in Uganda from their personal involvement with churches. CRANE is a network of Christian churches and projects in Kampala, Uganda. It is part of Viva, who build and support networks in a number of cities globally.

6. Toolkits and resources exist for guidance on the development of support groups such as Greg Satorie, *How to Start a Support Group* (Windhoek, Nambia: Catholic AIDS Action, 2003), Catholic AIDS Action, Namibia, and various resources of Strategies for Hope, http://www.strategiesforhope.org.

7. Rev. Isak P. Malua, participant at LUCSA workshop on Mainstreaming AIDS in Johannesburg, South Africa, 2010.

8. Paula Clifford, *Theology and the HIV/AIDS Epidemic*, Christian AID (August 2004), http://www.christianaid.org.uk/images/hiv_theologyfinal.pdf. Clifford cites Mary Garvey, *Dying to Learn: Young People, HIV and the Churches* (London: Christian Aid, 2003), and that book's foreword by Archbishop Njongonkulu Ndungane, Anglican Archbishop of Cape Town.

9. Solutions-focused (SF) therapy focuses on what clients want to achieve rather than on the problem(s) that made them to seek help. The approach does not focus on the past but, instead, focuses on the present and future. Believing that change is constant, the solution-focused leader or therapist helps people identify the things that they wish to have changed in their life and also to attend to those things that are currently happening that they wish to continue to have happen, SF therapists help their clients to construct a concrete vision of a *preferred future* for themselves. The process helps clients identify the skills, abilities, and external resources (e.g., social networks) that they already have and that identify them as competent individuals, and it also aims to help the client identify new ways of bringing these resources to bear upon the problem. Resources can be *internal*, concerning the client's skills, strengths, qualities, beliefs that are useful to them and their capacities; or *external*, focused on supportive relationships such as partners, family, friends, faith or religious groups, and also support groups.

10. Rachel Mash, Roselyn Kareithi, and Bob Mash, "Survey of Sexual Behaviour among Anglican Youth in the Western Cape," *South African Medical Journal* 96, no. 2 (2006): 124–27.

11. Jeanne Rogge Steel, "Teenage Sexuality and Media Practice: Factoring in the Influences of Family, Friends and School," *The Journal of Sex Research* 36, no. 4 (1999): 331–41.

12. Eileen Zurbriggen, et al., *Report of the APA Task Force on the Sexualization of Girls* (Washington, DC: American Psychological Association, 2007). http://www.apa.org/pi/women/programs/girls/report.aspx.

13. Ibid., 12, quoting D. Merskin, "Reviving Lolita? A Media Literacy Examination of Sexual Portrayals of Girls in Fashion Advertising," *American Behavioral Scientist* 48 (2004): 120.

14. Deborah L. Tolman and Emily A. Impett, "Looking Good, Sounding Good: Femininity Ideology and Adolescent Girls' Mental Health," *Psychology of Women Quarterly* 30 (2006): 85–95.

15. Street Child Africa, http://www.streetchildafrica.org.uk/pages/research-and-resources.html.

16. Avert, "Preventing Mother-to-Child Transmission (PMTCT) in Practice," http://www.avert.org/pmtct-hiv.htm.

17. Andrew Doupe, *Partnerships between Churches and People Living with HIV/AIDS Organisations* (Geneva: WCC Publications, 2006).

18. David Murrow, *Why Men Hate Going to Church* (Nashville: Thomas Nelson, 2005).

19. "Men of Quality Are Not Afraid of Equality," Padare/Enkundleni/Men's Forum on Gender, Harare, Zimbabwe, 2009.

20. Njuguna Thuka, "Still at Large," in *Defying the Odds: Lessons Learnt from Men for Gender Equity Now* (Nairobi, Kenya: FEMNET, 2012), http://femnet.co/index.php/en/component/k2/item/109-defying-the-odds-lessons-learnt-from-men-for-gender-equality-now.

21. Kennedy Odhiambo Otina, coordinator, 2004–2008, Men for Gender Equity Now (MEGEN), "The Emergence of a Men's Movement," in ibid., 13.

22. Ecumenical HIV & AIDS Initiative in Africa (EHAIA), a programme of the World Council of Churches, http://www.oikoumene.org/en/what-we-do/hivaids-initiative-in-africa.

23. Adapted from Nyambura Njoroge, *EHAIA Initiative in Africa Annual Review 2011* (Geneva: World Council of Churches, 2011).

24. Hazel Nyere Gutu and Ezra Chitando, *Transformative Masculinity* (Geneva: World Council of Churches, 2012).

25. Worldwide Marriage Encounter: http://www.wwme.org; Engagement Encounter: http://www.engagedencounter.org/infoseek.asp.

26. Patricia Love and Jo Robinson, *Hot Monogamy: Essential Steps to More Passionate, Intimate Lovemaking* (New York: Plume, 1995)

27. Bill and Pam Farrel, *Red-Hot Monogamy: Making Your Marriage Sizzle* (Eugene, OR: Harvest House, 2006).

28. http://www.africafatherhood.co.za/.

29. World YWCA, "Reducing the Risk of HIV Infection," May 2012, http://www.worldywca.org/YWCA-News/World-YWCA-and-Member-Associations-News/Reducing-the-risk-of-HIV-infection.

30. Source: United Nations Enable, http://www.un.org/disabilities.

31. World Council of Churches, "A Church of All and for All," interim statement presented to the 2003 WCC Central Committee Meeting, http://www.oikoumene. org/en/resources/documents/wcc-commissions/faith-and-order-commission/ ix-other-study-processes/a-church-of-all-and-for-all-an-interim-statement.

32. Ronald Nikkel, "Beyond Tolerance," *Conversatio Morum: Thoughts for a Monday Morning*, Prison Fellowship International, Toronto, October 2006, http://www.pfi.org/media-and-news/publications/CM023Oct06/view.

33. Donald E. Messer, "God So Loved the World," sermon for Trinity Sunday, 20/05/12, CABSA, http://www.cabsa.org.za/content/god-so-loved-world.

34. Recollections of Dr. Sue Parry from her 2003 fact-finding tour on the responses of faith-based organizations to HIV in Madagascar.

35. Message from the Pre-Assembly of People Living with HIV to the 13th General Assembly of Conference of Churches of Asia, Kuala Lumpur, 2011.

36. Definition adapted from Wikipedia, 2012, http://en.wikipedia.org/wiki/Support_group.

37. Daniel G Karslake, *For the Bible Tells Me So* (New York: FirstRunFeatures, 2007), documentary, 98 min., http://www.forthebibletellsmeso.org/indexd.htm.

38. Pope John Paul II, address given at Mission Dolores, 1987. Also see: Pope John Paul II, Tanzania, September 1990; Pope John Paul II, Burundi, September 1990; and in *The Church Responds to HIV/AIDS: A Caritas Internationalis Dossier*, ed. Duncan MacLaren (London: CAFOD, 1996).

39. Sue Parry, *Beacons of Hope: HIV Competent Churches—A Framework for Action.* (Geneva: WCC Publications, 2008).

40. "Framework for Engagement"—Greater participation of people living with HIV and AIDS in the life of the church, http://www.wcc-coe.org/wcc/what/mission/m-epub.html.

41. EMPACT Africa is a nonprofit organization, based in Austin, Texas, dedicated to helping local church leaders in southern Africa fight the stigma of HIV and AIDS in their congregations and communities. Dr. David Barstow is president of the EMPACT board.

42. Canon Gideon Byamugisha was the first religious leader to state openly his HIV-positive status. He has been living positively for over 20 years and was the founder of ANERELA+. He has been hugely instrumental in breaking down and challenging stigma, discrimination, action, and misaction toward people living with HIV.

43. World Bank, AIDS Campaign Team for Africa (ACTafrica), "Mainstreaming HIV/AIDS in Non-Health Operations in Sub-Saharan Africa: A User-Friendly Task Team Guide," December 2009, http://go.worldbank.org/3THFYO7EO0.

44. UNAIDS, "2004 Report on the Global AIDS Epidemic," http://data.unaids.org/Global-Reports/Bangkok-2004/unaidsbangkokpress/gar2004html/gar2004_00_en.htm.

45. Avert, "HIV Prevention Strategies," http://www.avert.org/abc-hiv.htm.

46. Christian AID, "HIV Is a Virus," http://www.christianaid.org.uk/images/HIVSAVELeaflet2010.pdf.

47. Scientific trials have shown that male circumcision can reduce the risk of a man becoming infected with HIV during heterosexual intercourse by up to 60 percent. These findings have led the World Health Organization and UNAIDS to recommend circumcision as an important element of HIV prevention. See UNAIDS 2011 World AIDS Day Report, http://www.unaids.org/en/resources/publications/2011/name,63525,en.asp.

48. INERELA+, "What Is SAVE?," http://www.focagifo.org/downloads/what-is-save.pdf.

49. World Health Organization (WHO), "Guidance on Provider Initiated HIV Counselling and Testing in Health Facilities," WHO/UNAIDS, May 2007, http://www.who.int/hiv/pub/vct/pitc2007/en/.

50. World Health Organization (WHO), "Guidance on Couples HIV Testing and Counselling (CHTC)," WHO/UNAIDS, April 2012, http://www.who.int/hiv/pub/guidelines/9789241501972/en/.

51. Reflections from Dr. Sue Parry after exposure visit to numerous HIV-competent programmes in Karnataka State, India, 2010.

52. Dr. Kevin de Cock, director of WHO's Department of HIV/AIDS commenting on the ARHAP report, *Appreciating Assets: The Contribution of Religion to Universal Access in Africa*, http://www.arhap.uct.ac.za/downloads/ARHAPWHO_execsumm.pdf.

53. Nancy S. Padian, et al., "The Future of HIV Prevention," *Journal of Acquired Immune Deficiency Syndrome* 60, Supplement 2 (August 2012): S22–26.

54. ARHAP, *Appreciating Assets: The Contribution of Religion to Universal Access in Africa*, http://www.arhap.uct.ac.za/downloads/ARHAPWHO_execsumm.pdf.

55. Ecumenical Pharmaceutical Network (EPN), *HIV & AIDS Treatment Literacy Guide for Church Leaders*, 2010, http://www.epnetwork.org/hiv-treatment-literacy-manual.

56. Debbie DeVoe, "Churches Become HIV Clinics in South Africa," Catholic Relief Services, http://crs.org/south-africa/art-transition-tour/.

57. Ibid.

58. UNAIDS, "2006 Report on the Global AIDS Epidemic," http://www.who.int/hiv/mediacentre/news60/en/.

59. United Nations Children's Fund (UNICEF), *PMTCT Report Card 2005: Monitoring Progress on the Implementation of Programs to Prevent Mother-to-Child Transmission of HIV* (New York: UNICEF, 2005).

60. World Health Organization (WHO)/United Nations Population Fund (UNFPA), "Glion Consultation on Strengthening the Linkages between Reproductive Health and HIV/AIDS: Family Planning and HIV/AIDS in Women and Children," 2006, http://www.who.int/reproductivehealth/publications/family_planning/HIV_06_2/en/index.html.

61. Marie-Louise Newella, et al., "Mortality of Infected and Uninfected Infants Born to HIV-Infected Mothers in Africa: A Pooled Analysis," *Lancet* 364, no. 9441 (2004): 1236–243.

62. UNAIDS, "The Religious Community Working towards Zero New HIV Infections among Children," 13 April 2012, http://www.cabsa.org.za/content/religious-community-working-towards-zero-new-hiv-infections-among-children-13412.

63. Robin Root, "'That's When Life Changed': Client Experiences of Church Run Home-based Care in Swaziland," A report for the Health Economics and HIV/AIDS Division (HEARD), University of KwaZulu-Natal, October 2011, http://www.shbcare.org/docs/Ch.urchRunHBC.HEARD.Root.pdf.

64. Weddy Silomba, "HIV/AIDS and Development: The Chikankata Experience," Paper prepared for United Nations Research Institute for Social Development (UNRISD) project on HIV/AIDS Development, Zambia, 2002, http://www.unrisd.org/80256B3C005BCCF9/%28httpPublications%29/D610492CF61A089CC1256BB8004FC346?OpenDocument.

65. Diocese of False Bay in the Anglican Church of Southern Africa, http://www.falsebaydiocese.org.za/projects.

66. Mashambanzou Care Trust, http://www.mashambanzou.co.zw/.

67. Ronald Nikkel, "A Redemption Story," *Conversatio Morum: Thoughts for a Monday Morning*, Prison Fellowship International, 23 April 2012, http://www.pfi.org/media-and-news/publications/a-redemption-story/view?searchterm=A%20Redemption%20Story.

68. United Nations Office on Drugs and Crime (UNODC), "Exclusion Is Not an Option: Turning the HIV Tide in Prisons," June 2012.

69. Prison Fellowship International, "Church Engagement: An Introduction," http://www.pfi.org/cot/church.

70. UNAIDS, *Report on the Global AIDS Epidemic 2010*, http://www.unaids.org/globalreport/global_report.htm.

71. UNAIDS, "2011 UN Political Declaration on HIV/AIDS—Targets and elimination commitments," in *Global AIDS Response Progress Reporting 2013: Construction of Core Indicators for monitoring the 2011 UN Political Declaration on HIV/AIDS*, (Geneva: UNAIDS, 2013), 8, http://www.unaids.org/en/media/unaids/contentassets/documents/document/2013/GARPR_2013–guidelines_en.pdf.

72. Leigh Price, et al., "Zimbabwean Stories of 'Best Practice' in Mitigating the HIV Crisis through a Cultural and Gender Perspective," Changing the River's Flow series, SAfAIDS, Harare, March 2009, http://www.safaids.net/files/Changing%20river%20Best%20Practice.pdf.

73. Ann Veneman, Executive Director, UNICEF, http://www.arcapartners.org/hivaids.cfm.

74. Ndunge Kiiti, et al. "Conceptualizing and Measuring Empowerment," oral presentation, Oxford Round Table, Oxford, UK, August, 2008; Monique Hennink, et al. "Defining Empowerment: Perspectives from Developmental Organisations," Development in Practice 22, no. 2 (April 2012): 202–15.

75. Parry, *Beacons of Hope*.

76. Diocese of False Bay in the Anglican Church of Southern Africa, http://www.falsebaydiocese.org.za/projects.

77. Parry, *Beacons of Hope*.

Section 9. Stewarship of Time, Talents, Finances, and Resources

1. Mark Dybul, Peter Piot, and Julio Frenk, "Reshaping Global Health," *Policy Review* 173 (June 2012), http://www.hoover.org/publications/policy-review/article/118116.

Section 10. Monitoring, Evaluation, and Knowledge Sharing

1. NGO Code of Good Practice, "Self-Assessment Checklist: Mainstreaming HIV," http://www.hivcode.org.

2. Sue Holden, *Mainstreaming HIV/AIDS in Development and Humanitarian Programmes* (Oxford: Oxfam GB/ActionAid/Save the Children UK, 2004).

3. Carter McNamara, "Basic Guide to Outcome-Based Evaluation for Nonprofit Organizations with Very Limited Resources," adapted from *Field Guide to Nonprofit Program Design, Marketing and Evaluation*, 4th ed. (Minneapolis: Authenticity Consulting, L.L.C., 2002, 2006).

4. Sue Parry, *Beacons of Hope: HIV Competent Churches—A Framework for Action* (Geneva: WCC Publications, 2008).

Conclusion

1. Fr. Robert Igo, OSB, Christ the Word Monastery, Macheke, Zimbabwe (2009).